Howard Hiatt

Howard Hiatt

How This Extraordinary Mentor Transformed Health with Science and Compassion

Mark Rosenberg

The MIT Press
Cambridge, Massachusetts
London, England

This book was set in Stone Serif by Westchester Publishing Services.

Library of Congress Cataloging-in-Publication Data
Names: Rosenberg, Mark L., 1945– author.
Title: Howard Hiatt : how this extraordinary mentor transformed health with science and compassion / Mark Rosenberg ; foreword by Michelle A. Williams.
Description: Cambridge, MA : The MIT Press, [2018] | Includes index.
Identifiers: LCCN 2018007482 | ISBN 9780262038805 (hardcover : alk. paper), ISBN 9780262546690 (paperback)
Subjects: | MESH: Hiatt, Howard H. | Harvard School of Public Health. | Schools, Public Health--history | Physicians--history | Public Health--history | History, 20th Century | United States | Biography
Classification: LCC R747.H28 | NLM WZ 100 | DDC 610.71/17444--dc23
    LC record available at https://lccn.loc.gov/2018007482

Contents

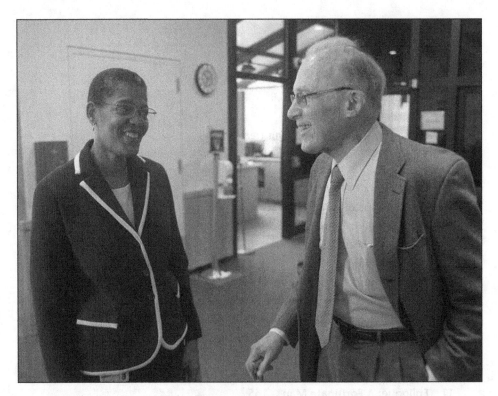

Two deans, Michelle Williams and Howard Hiatt, with tenures separated by more than four decades, met in 2018 and found they shared similar hopes and aspirations for the Harvard-Chan School of Public Health and global health broadly. (Photograph by Kent Dayton.)

Foreword

Public health, an inherently multidisciplinary field, has seen many champions, of various educational and professional backgrounds, whose names and legacies are forever linked with not only the institutions they served, but also the people they affected through their ideas, work, and mentorship. With an impressive career spanning six decades, Dr. Howard Hiatt is undoubtedly one of these champions of public health, a remarkable physician, scholar, academic leader, mentor, and teacher. Howard's leadership of the then-Harvard School of Public Health enabled it to thrive. While his ideas were not immediately embraced, he has made a lasting impact on public health, in this institution and globally.

Howard Hiatt was a leader ahead of his time who championed change in challenging times for the Harvard School of Public Health. Prior to his appointment as dean, the School was underperforming according to the university's standards, both academically and financially. Derek Bok, Harvard's president at the time, was considering three options with respect to the school: close it down, merge it with the medical school, or bring leadership that could turn it around. He entrusted the school to Dr. Hiatt, a leading molecular biologist and a distinguished clinician and research scholar, who prior to that was the first Blumgart Professor of Medicine at Harvard Medical School and Physician-in-Chief at Beth Israel Hospital. Howard was Bok's first decanal appointee, chosen after much reflection and with a strong mandate for change to improve the school's academic standards and modernize its curriculum. Serving as dean from 1972 to 1984, Howard brought creative, visionary leadership, which was essential to repositioning the school. As he said in an interview with the *Boston Globe* in 2013, he "brought a lot of what had never been in a school of public health."

At the time when his deanship began, the field of public health did not have the standing it has in the public's mind today. It was before the HIV/AIDS epidemic and before the investments of major funders of global health programs like the Bill and Melinda Gates Foundation elevated the importance of health and made it a priority in the development and human rights agendas. As a prominent representative of the medical field, Howard was commited to enhance visibility to public health, which earned instant respect to that field in medicine. He saw public health as the best vector for joining his interest in medicine with his passion for improving health and equity at the population level. Ironically, the fact that he did not have a public health background was one of the reasons for resentment by some of the faculty at the School of Public Health.

Since he had been educated in medicine, and not public health, at the start of his deanship Howard devoted several months to learning about the field and studying the curricula in public health at Harvard and other universities. That thread of continuous learning has been present throughout his life. The value of Howard's forward-thinking approach can be seen in some of the first statements he made as an incumbent dean. In a 1972 interview with the *Harvard Crimson*, he spoke of "a distortion of priorities in the health fields," citing the "emphasis placed on curative medicine rather than in areas of prevention." He underlined the necessity for health and medical professionals to concentrate more on disease prevention—a popular concept in both public health and medicine today. He also foresaw "great opportunities to work with people in state and municipal agencies in planning effective health programs."

Howard's deanship was a period of rapid fermentation and change at the School of Public Health. He started with energy, commitment, and a real sense of mission to innovate the curriculum. He brought in world-class scientists and new faculty members with areas of expertise that were not represented at the school. Under his leadership, the school's biostatistics programs and quantitative analytic work were strengthened, molecular and cell biology were introduced into its teaching and research, and the preceding department of health services administration was modernized to become the first public health school program in health policy and management. Howard was keen on innovative cross-faculty programs before those were fashionable in academia. During his deanship, the School of Public Health organized seminar discussions inviting faculty from many parts of Harvard, including its schools of medicine, law, government, public health, and business. Ideas and expertise were exchanged, and key figures were recruited to the school through these discussions.

Howard's experience offers valuable lessons for current leaders of the best schools of public health, and indeed, of any healthcare organization. Some of the key priorities of his deanship are strikingly similar to my own agenda forty-five years later. He focused on many areas that we still prioritize in our work, such as understanding and working closely with the surrounding community in order to improve its well-being; strengthening public health as a movement to promote equity and better health and heathcare for all; emphasizing the quantitative and qualitative analytical tools and skills that can be used to improve the healthcare system, improve health outcomes, and lower costs; and fostering interdisciplinary collaborations to address current and future health challenges. With these ambitious goals, Howard took the school in new and innovative directions, bringing its public health education to a more advanced level. A *Boston Globe* article noted in 1978 that he "had forged strong beginnings of programs aimed at training 'new kinds of public health professionals' with expertise in other fields, such as law, economics, engineering, business, and social and environmental sciences."

As shown in this book, Howard's deanship was an incredibly difficult time for him because of the resistance to change that he encountered at the School of Public Health. The conflict with senior faculty made headlines in the *Boston Globe* and the *New York Times*. But Howard's passionate efforts were not in vain, as he and the key recruitments he made were able to truly transform the institution. His values and ideas, once accepted, have become integral to the fabric of the school. They have been shared and built on by his successors, including myself. The school has continued to evolve, and today it is stronger for Howard's fortitude, vision, commitment, and leadership.

Since I became dean of the recently renamed Harvard T.H. Chan School of Public Health, my aspiration has been to sustain and build on the excellence in education, research, and leadership that the institution has exemplified over the past century. It is a privilege to be the fifth dean after Howard. It is because of him and his eminent successors that this excellence has been achieved, and thanks to them, the school community continues to pursue novel and integrated ways to address the most pressing issues in global public health.

Howard's distinguished career has continued for decades since he left the School of Public Health with many notable achievements. He spearheaded the Program in Clinical Effectiveness, a joint initiative of two hospitals and Harvard's medical and public health schools, which has been called a jewel in the crown of the university. As a fantastic tool for enabling the brightest clinicians to obtain training in fundamental analytic techniques and perspectives on how to drive and manage change in healthcare organizations, the program has been a dramatic success.

As a cofounder and associate chief of Brigham and Women's Hospital's Division of Global Health Equity, Howard has continued to advocate on behalf of vulnerable populations in the United States and around the world. He helped create a first-of-its-kind physician training program in global health, and as Paul Farmer put it, built "a new medical field from scratch." The division has been attracting extraordinary young people as global health residents, and it has become a model for other academic medical institutions. In Howard's words reflected in his 2013 interview with the *Boston Globe*, "It has opened a whole new area, a commitment on the part of this major teaching hospital, this major medical school, this major organization called Partners in Health, to the problems of impoverished people throughout the world."

Early on in his career, Howard became aware of the importance of finding a great mentor. He credits his first mentor with opening his eyes to "what science meant, what it could be," and how to ask meaningful questions and seek answers. In turn, Howard has always been a champion of young and rising professionals and scholars. From the time he was the chief of residents at Beth Israel Hospital, he has been interested in the constant career development of young people, and he has trained and mentored thousands of physicians and medical students. Dr. Harvey Fineberg, Howard's successor as dean, underlined Howard's "career-long emphasis on the next generation: through personal mentorship of individuals, but also reflected in the values he held around education." Among Harvey's fondest memories of his mentor are the gatherings Howard and his late wife Doris hosted at their home. Harvey loved those informal events, as they were excellent opportunities to interact with colleagues. These occasions influenced his own thinking to work closely with the next generation as he embarked on his own illustrious career in medicine and public health.

This book is a labor of love by another of Howard's distinguished mentees. The author, Dr. Mark Rosenberg, worked for twenty years with the

Centers for Disease Control and Prevention, and served for sixteen years as president of the Task Force for Global Heath, a nonprofit organization dedicated to building coalitions to promote global health and human development. The author leads readers along the journey and learning path that Howard Hiatt followed, distilling his mentor's experience and telling the story interwoven with views from Howard's personal memoir and quotes from his contemporaries, as a way to bring readers to a deeper understanding of the real person, the mentor, the leader.

I share the gratitude of Howard's many students, mentees, and colleagues, for his vision, the knowledge and lessons he has given to all of us, and the appreciation he has instilled in us for the importance of rigorous science and life-long learning. Howard's role as a teacher and adviser to many professionals in medicine and public health, including influential figures like Paul Farmer, Jim Yong Kim, Don Berwick, Harvey Fineberg, Milton Weinstein, William (Bill) Hsiao, and Mark Rosenberg, is an inseparable and rewarding part of his wonderful legacy.

In a thorough and engaging way, this biography also offers a fascinating insight into the complexity and challenge of leadership—not only leadership in public health and medicine, but leadership in general. In order to lead and improve complex organizations, one has to be an agent of change. What does it take to be an effective leader? What is the personal price you pay when faced with opposition to change? What capabilities does one need to manage a complex institution? This book presents the true and quite remarkable story of a man—kind, caring, and extremely accomplished, with a brilliant mind and vision— who introduced major changes in several medical and public health institutions. In doing so, he significantly improved them, thus ensuring that they met society's expectations—to educate health professionals with the variety of skills they need and to be strong advocates of health promotion and better healthcare for people everywhere.

Michelle Williams
Dean of the Faculty, Harvard T.H. Chan School of Public Health

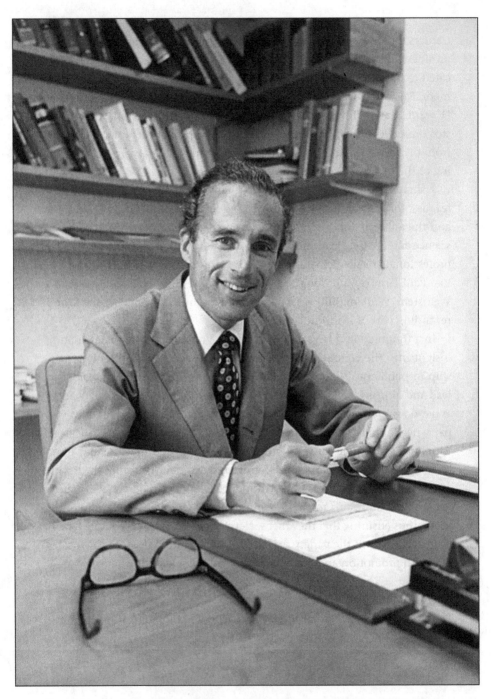

Howard in the dean's office at the Harvard School of Public Health in 1976. (Photograph by Mark Rosenberg.)

Preface

Howard Hiatt had been a wonderful mentor and friend for almost forty years when we first discussed writing a book together. When we first started to talk about it, in October 2010, Howard asked me to remind him how we first got together. I emailed him back that "I think I first started to hear about you during our second year of medical school, when I was working on some of the anti-war protests and on trying to get a neighborhood voice into the discussion about building the 'new' Affiliated Hospitals complex in Mission Hill. I think it was when Harvey and I were living together on Mission Hill that we invited you and Doris for dinner. We decided to invite the faculty member we would most like to know. A few years later you made it possible for me to do the *Patients* book and gave me a position at HSPH when Jill and I moved back from Atlanta to Boston in 1976. And then many things and many people drew us closer."

When we began to work on this book, nine years ago, my goal was to help Howard write a book that he wanted to write about how he had tried to bring about change in three different medical institutions with three different outcomes. I wanted to help him because he had, over many years, done so much to help me. It soon became clear that his experience at the second of these three institutions—as dean of the Harvard School of Public Health—had been terribly painful and that writing this book could be a way to help him get past that pain and see his life as a much more positive whole, an arc bending toward social justice and compassion. I sent him this email:

Rosenberg, Mark rosenberg@taskforce.org 12/27/10

To: Howard, PJaneway

Hi Howie,

I just wanted to mention some of the important things that our conversation got me thinking about (in no particular order):

1. It might be useful to just list all the memories you have—don't censor anything out—and then figure out how you might use them or draw lessons from them. And how you want to organize them. Don't demand from yourself that the organization of the material must come to you at the same time that you remember the different items.

2. Tracey Kidder suffered mightily and for a long time he was depressed after he had collected and written down all his material for *Mountains Beyond Mountains.* The way to organize the material was the hardest part of the book for him.

3. The three dimensions of change—rational (ideas/science/policy), institutional, and personal—are all very important parts of your journey. I think this might be one useful set of categories for describing the types of change you brought about at the different places you worked. I would not discount or short-change any of these areas.

4. I think you are most comfortable and have brought about enormous changes in ideas and thinking, in the science of public health. You have also brought about significant changes in the organizations you have worked with. I think you might be least comfortable with the personal changes and the emotional/psychological change that has been part of your journey. But sometimes the area we are least comfortable with is the richest area to mine.

5. You were a great mentor while you were at the BI, but you became a spectacular mentor after the HSPH experience. Your relationship with my brothers, Don, Paul, and Jim, and myself is probably more intense and qualitatively different from the mentoring relationships you had earlier. I think that the HSPH experience had something to do with this scaling up in intensity.

Well, it turned out to be a beginning, for sure, but we would never have guessed that it would take eight years to get to the finish. And it turned out not to be one person's race against time, but a relay in which different people would carry the baton. While I have been part of the team and ran the last leg of the race, it has truly been a team effort. I have relied heavily on parts of the memoir that Howard and Penny Janeway wrote together, *Making Change,* and I am indebted to Howard and Penny. They and I spent many hours, days, and weeks trying to organize the vast amount of material, people and events that Howard remembered. Several different authors offered to help us with the writing, but when none worked out, Howard and Penny put together a memoir, which was quite a complete compilation of all that Howard remembered and had documented. It is accessible on the MIT Press website [https://mitpress.mit.edu/books/howard-hiatt] for anyone who would like to know more details.

Howard's memoir is comprehensive and long but it did not really tell his story. We were very fortunate to find a wonderful writer and human being in Charlie Kenney, who helped to transform a large part of the memoir—and much more—into a real story. I cannot overstate the importance of Charlie's contributions to this book. He interviewed Howard and many people who had worked closely with Howard for a long time. He is the consummate professional, and I benefited from his skills and experience as he encouraged me and coached me. Without Charlie's help this book would not exist. I owe him more than I can say.

I also want to thank Derek Bok, former president of Harvard University, and Howard's brother, Arnie Hiatt, who were generous with their time, and thoughtful and honest in their interviews. I am also grateful to Harvey Fineberg, who succeeded Howard as dean of the Harvard School of Public Health, then crossed the Charles River and went on to become provost of Harvard University, then president of the Institute of Medicine, and finally president and CEO of the Gordon and Betty Moore Foundation. My thanks to Harvey for the generous financial support that the Moore Foundation provided. Additional information in this book came from interviews that were generously given by many individuals, including Tony Komoroff, Milt Weinstein, Bill Hsaio, Anne Nicholson, Joel Katz, Wilbert Jordan, and Marshall Wolf.

Important information about Global Health at Home came from Sonya Shin and Heidi Behforouz via the Washington Global Health Alliance and the program Global2Local. Adam Taylor, Lisa Cohen, David Fleming, and Tina Vlasaty were wonderful colleagues in helping Howard, Charlie Kenney, and me put together the conference on this subject at the Institute for Healthcare Improvement where Maureen Bisangnano, Don Berwick, Don Goldman, and Pamela Arndt worked hard to make it happen.

Jon Rosenberg was extremely generous with his editorial assistance in putting together the article "Global Health at Home: Harvesting Innovations from around the World to Improve American Medical Care" that appeared in *Harvard Magazine* (November–December 2016) and served as a basis for chapter 9 of this book.

I am deeply grateful to my brothers Jim Kim, Paul Farmer, and Don Berwick for their interviews, encouragement, continuing friendship, and inspiring leadership in creating their own paths for making this world better for the poorest and most vulnerable people on this planet.

Barbara Rosen has worked closely with Howard at the Brigham and Women's Hospital for twenty-three years and has helped us communicate, get information, get photographs, and get through cloudy days with her optimism and wonderful caring. I am also grateful to my daughter Julie for many things, and specifically for always being available even late at night to walk me through technical glitches with one or more of the electronic tools that befuddle me.

Lindsay Morrisey, the program coordinator for the program in clinical effectiveness at the Brigham and Women's Hospital, and Susan Pasternak of the Beth Israel Deaconness Medical Archives were extremely helpful in tracking down photographs of Howard Hiatt when he worked at the Harvard Hospitals. And Cathy Pate, the Brigham and Womens' Hospital archivist also worked for the Center for the History of Medicine at the Francis A. Countway Library of Medicine and her colleague Jack Flagler helped us search the Harvard Medical School archives for photographs and other relevant documents. Michelle Williams took time from her packed-full and demanding schedule to read the manuscript carefully, understand the parallels between two deans forty-four years apart, and write a terrific foreword that made their connections clear and compelling. Kathryn Galvin helped to make this possible and helped to get a photograph of these two deans together.

There were many other people who have known Howard and supported him. I could not include everyone, but I hope they do understand that Howard appreciates them all.

Any mistakes or errors that are in this book are solely my responsibility and I apologize for any errors of omission or commission.

While this book began as the story of Howard's experience at three medical and public health institutions, it ended up as a much larger story, the story of Howard Hiatt's life. And for me it turned into a much larger undertaking than I had ever anticipated. It took much more time and required more struggles than I planned—at the beginning—to give. But our lives don't follow plans. Neither do books. And through it all, my wonderful wife Jill provided support, sustenance, and the sanity I sometimes struggled to find.

Introduction: A Thank You from Our Hearts

One day when one of us was out with his grandson who was just about to turn six, the young man asked, "Poppi, do you know what the best thing about being a kid is?" His grandfather said "no, tell me." And he responded, "OK, Poppi, the best thing about being a kid is that you still have so far to go before you die." His grandfather turned the question around, and asked the boy if he knew what was the best thing about being old. "No, Poppi, I am only five." "The best thing about being old," the grandfather answered, "is that you have learned a lot of lessons and you get to share them with the people you love."

Howard Hiatt has learned a lot of lessons in his ninety-three years, and he has never stopped sharing them with the people he loves. Indeed, we see that as the central goal of this book: to share his lessons with all of those he loves ... and with many more. As recipients and beneficiaries of his generosity of spirit, we are deeply grateful. We have also benefited by his having brought the four of us together, first as colleagues, now as friends, to the point where we refer to ourselves as "the four brothers." We are also grateful for the appreciation he has instilled in us for science and continuous learning. At ninety-three, he is still actively learning. His life is testament to a wonderful combination of learning, giving, and loving. That reveals itself as mentoring.

Neither work nor life is easy. We wish we could control our future and try to be thoughtful in our choices. But sooner or later we learn that life doesn't go according to any plan. Wonderful opportunities arise that we never imagined we would be able to take advantage of, and so do problems—surprisingly many of them. A mentor can comfort us in helping us deal with these problems. For each of us, Howard Hiatt has done that.

Howard also showed us something that they never taught us in school about being happy. In school, the emphasis was always: "If you want to be happy, you need to do well on your PSATs, SATs, MCATs; excel in college, pick the right major and excel in it while maintaining a high overall GPA; get into the right medical school; do well on your boards; get the right recommendations for residency; pick the right specialty; get the right residency; get the right job; and then, finally, you will be happy." But although we have lived between fifty-eight and seventy-three years now, it took each of us a good many years before we realized that the most important determinant of whether we will be happy at work is not those achievement tests or other external measures of accomplishment, but rather the *people* we work with. Happiness depends on whether they respect us and our values, and whether we share their values, and how they treat people. Howard modeled that kind of person for us.

For each of us, it required an active decision to get to know Howard and establish a relationship with him. The great American author, Philip Roth, found his mentor in his high school English teacher, Bob. Roth wrote a book about "how to become ... a bold and honorable and effective man. This is no easy task," he wrote, in talking about his mentor, "for there are ... one's massive imperfections of intelligence, emotion, foresight and judgment." We are all, each and every one of us, so far from perfect in our intelligence, emotion, foresight, and judgment. Over the years Roth had many conversations with Bob. Roth realized that our education goes on over the course of our whole life, and a good mentor he thought was so very important, not just "to a boy's but to an adult's education: in loss, grief and, that inescapable component of living, betrayal."[1] And most important, Roth wrote about himself and his mentor: "I will put the matter in plain language, directly as I can: I believe we fell in love with each other." We, too, have been fortunate to fall in love with an extraordinary mentor. What rare and truly wonderful luck!

There is a connection between having a mentor and finding happiness. In 2010, two Harvard psychologists, Matthew Killingsworth and Daniel Gilbert, performed a study that used an iPhone app to ask volunteers, at random moments, what they were doing and how happy they were. They discovered that we spend most of our lives not thinking about what we are doing at that moment, whether it's shopping, eating or, in particular, working. No matter how enjoyable the activity, this gift for distraction comes at a psychic cost: "a wandering mind," they wrote in the journal *Science*, "is an unhappy mind." In a modern world, when can we come closest to our original, thought-free happiness? Well, the Harvard psychologists noted that, besides sex, the two activities during which we are most fully in the present are conversation and exercise. A mentor is someone you converse with, really talk to, and really connect with. That is the beauty and joy of it. For each of us, Howard Hiatt has been such a very special person.

When you get a chance to examine the life of a mentor, it starts to look much more like a real life, the kind of life we know, the kind that goes with real human beings. Howard's life, like all lives, has not always been easy, not always happy. In his story that follows you will get an idea of what he has done, and how he has persevered. Howard found the qualities he may have missed in his father in a warm and supportive mentor of his own. And Howard became an extraordinary mentor himself, a teacher and boss who led by giving praise and support. But when asked by the president of Harvard to take on the role of dean and fix a school of public health that was not up to the university's standards, he met fierce opposition to the changes he wanted to bring. Those changes would make a great agenda for change today even at the very best schools of public health:

- Improve the quantitative and qualitative analytical tools and skills that can be used to improve the health care system, improve health, and lower costs.
- Support the type of interdisciplinary collaboration that is needed to solve the most important health and public health problems facing us today and in the near future.
- Understand and work closely with your community to understand its problems, mobilize resources, and improve its health and well-being.
- Recognize that we share this planet with many low- and middle-income countries that have a lot to teach us and where working together can be mutually beneficial.
- Mobilize the power of global health with not only the tools needed, but with the moral and ethical values needed to address health inequities.
- Stand up for the values of public health.

Howard's ambitious approach was occasionally met with resistance by some faculty. So, after serving as dean for ten years, he left the school of public health—having largely succeeded but at a significant personal toll—and returned to teaching and supporting young physicians and health professionals. Through this whole process he became a mentor extraordinaire and found satisfaction in mentoring many more generations of young people who shared his same zeal to fix medicine and improve health around the world. He continues that work to this day.

We thank Howard from the bottom of our hearts for being such an extraordinary mentor to us. We are delighted that this book may give readers a chance to be as lucky as we have been to learn from him and maybe even to pass along the gift of mentoring to future generations. There is an old African proverb: "If you want to go fast, go alone. If you want to go far, go together." Our shared experience of Howard teaches us that one of the most important choices you will ever make in the journey of life is choosing your guides and companions.

Don Berwick
Paul Farmer
Jim Yong Kim
Mark Rosenberg

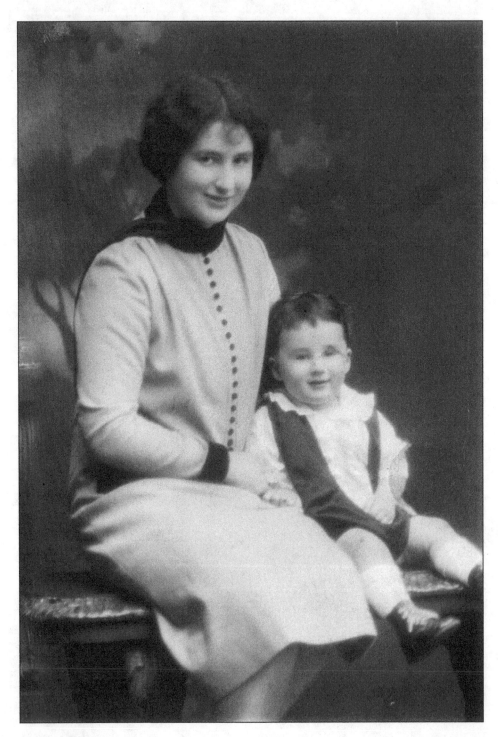

Figure 1.1
Howard with his mother, Dorothy.

1 What Kind of World Was This?

On a wintry day in 2016, Howard Hiatt makes his way through Harvard Yard, past John Harvard, the university founder seated comfortably in bronze, nicely weathering the years, much as his legacy weathers the centuries. The yard bustles, as always, with disheveled students, wide-eyed applicants on campus tours, and an array of preoccupied faculty. It is early February, seventy-four years almost to the day since Howard first walked this very pathway as a seventeen-year-old Harvard College freshman. On that day, he was a boundlessly energetic teenager with an outsized intellect and a determination to do something special with his life. Since then, much has changed and nothing has changed. Yes, he moves with greater care now that he has reached his tenth decade, not quite as certain in his stride. His memory falters now and again and the seven-plus decades have bent him slightly, weathered his lean, handsome visage. But the intellect is still immensely powerful as is his determination to do things that matter in the world. He passes Widener Library, one of the great collections on any campus worldwide. How many hours did he spend in Widener, in particular, as an undergraduate preparing for what lay ahead? Students spill out of Wigglesworth, a freshman dorm, as Howard completes his walk through the Yard and across Massachusetts Avenue, down Holyoke, a little side street, to Mt. Auburn St., where he turns right. He is not far from the red bricked Spee Club and or from the other exclusive private clubs—Fly, Owl, Porcellian (he was a member of none of these). Howard walks the few blocks west, past the Kennedy School of Government, to an elegant brick structure tucked away between Mt. Auburn and the Charles River. This tastefully designed condominium building, on what was Harvard property, is where Howard now resides. Fittingly, it is within steps of the campus.

During the nearly seven and a half decades since he first trod this path, Howard Hiatt has traveled the world, yet he has never been far from the hallowed academic ground of this university that he loves. Whether listening to the concerns of patients in Africa, Asia, South America, or elsewhere, he has remained tethered to this university. Whether treating an individual patient or conducting research destined to aid millions of patients, he has always done so as a son of Harvard. This place, and all of the intellectual rigor and passion for which, at its best, it stands, has defined Howard, just as he, in his way, has helped to define it.

It is ironic to consider that this lifelong relationship came perilously close to never happening. As he sits in his living room talking about that time so long ago, he recalls vividly the day he raced home from high school and found one of those thin envelopes, the kind universally dreaded by applicants. Howard was a beanpole of a seventeen-year-old when he read the letter informing him that he had *not* been admitted to Harvard College. He had felt certain he would be admitted, not based on any independent judgment of his own, but rather because of the assurance of Mr. Harold Fenner, principal at Classical High School in Worcester, Massachusetts. Mr. Fenner had all but guaranteed Howard that he would be admitted to Harvard. The valedictorian from Classical was nearly always admitted, said Mr. Fenner, and, though Howard was still in junior year, Mr. Fenner noted that based on academic standing Howard would surely earn that distinction upon graduation, and that he need apply nowhere other than Harvard.

There was something particularly stinging about the rejection. Howard's father had emigrated from Lithuania and neither he nor his young wife possessed much in the way of formal schooling. It was their dream that their children, Howard and his two younger siblings, gain the best possible education. Howard dreaded sharing the news with his parents. "For my father, Harvard was the glittering prize," Howard recalls. "A Harvard man was, for him, the elite of elites." In high school, when Howard asked permission to attend dancing class, his father took the matter under advisement and then reported back that permission was denied. He explained to Howard that he had consulted a man whose opinion he respected—a *Harvard man*, in fact—who advised against that form of recreation. Among his parents' most determined ambition was to find the finest educational pathway for their children, the classic immigrant impulse at the time. "Jewish parents look at the education of their children as a crucial matter," says Howard, "and for my parents, who had such limited education, they really expected that I would break out of that mold."

Howard's father, Alexander Chaitowicz, was barely fifteen years old when he left his home in the village of Obeliai, Lithuania, in search of opportunity in the new world. At Ellis Island Chaitowicz became Hiatt and young Al Hiatt went to a relative in Illinois, where he found work as a coal miner while he learned the language of his new country. Howard's mother, Dorothy Askinas, dropped out of high school in the third year to help support the family financially. Their pursuit of the American dream for their children was the classic immigrant aspirational story.

The day after receiving the letter of rejection, Howard went to the principal's office to see Mr. Fenner, who had no intention of letting this stand. In Howard's presence, Mr. Fenner phoned the director of admissions at Harvard and noted that the valedictorian at Classical had traditionally been welcomed at Harvard and he asked why Howard had not been admitted. And then Mr. Fenner posed a simple question: "Is it because this one is Jewish that you have turned him down?" He ended the conversation by saying that he would be in the admissions office the next morning.

This was 1942 in a world where manifestations of anti-Semitism were as varied as they were ubiquitous. There were personal rebukes—a man refusing to rent lakeside accommodations to Howard and his father because, he told them, they were Jewish. There was the boy in grade school who called Howard a "dirty Jew." ("Well, just avoid him," was his mother's counsel.)

And now Harvard. Throughout the 1920s and 1930s, as increasing numbers of Jewish students were admitted, a backlash among alumni grew. In 1925, an alum writing to the university's president expressed "fearful shock" that the university "had become so Hebrewized."[1] Blame for this trend rested with a standardized entrance examination on which many Jewish applicants performed well. Thus came the development of new admission guidelines—a more "holistic review," as it was described. Under this approach admission was based on more than a simple test metric. Whether one was a legacy, a "gentleman," or an accomplished athlete became legitimate criteria for admissions. Many decades later, writing in the *New York Times,* David Brooks observed that the Harvard provost "argued in several essays that Harvard did not want to become dominated by the 'sensitive, neurotic boy,' by those who are 'intellectually over-stimulated.' Instead, he said, Harvard should be seeking out boys who are of the 'healthy extrovert kind.' In 1950, Yale's president, A. Whitney Griswold, reassured alumni that the Yale man of the future would not be a 'beetle-browed, highly specialized intellectual, but a well-rounded man.' That year 278 students from elite prep schools applied to Harvard and 245 were accepted."[2]

There is a certain irony in all of this. In the twenty-first century a holistic review of Howard's application would have found that he was not only a brilliant student, but also had edited, written, and distributed the school magazine; had written and announced a weekly news radio program ("Youth Speaks") broadcast on a Worcester station; had worked Saturdays in his uncle's shoe store; and was considered a model leader by his high school faculty. In 1942, however, Howard was not seen in that rich context by Harvard.

The admission dean's response to Mr. Fenner's pointed question is lost to history. The day after that phone call, however, Mr. Fenner made his way the forty-four miles from Worcester to Cambridge and, days later, another letter arrived from Harvard with the joyful news that Howard was, in fact, admitted. Thus did seventeen-year-old Howard venture alone, by train, from Worcester to Boston and then on to Cambridge, where he arrived and entered Harvard in February 1943 and matriculated with the Harvard College class of 1946. Because there was a war going on, Howard's academic credentials were strong enough to let him begin at Harvard midway through his senior year in high school. Technically, he would not graduate from Classical High until June of that year, while well into his freshman year at Harvard, and he would return to deliver the valedictory address at Classical as a college student. On the day he arrived in Cambridge, Howard's life changed. He had never set foot on the Harvard campus before. In a way, over the coming seven decades, he would never leave.

Harvard has been central to Howard's life from the day he entered the college and remained so right up to his tenth decade. He has been an undergraduate, a student in the school of medicine, tenured professor in the medical school, chief of medicine at a major Harvard teaching hospital, dean of the school of public health, and cofounder of a major new division at another Harvard teaching hospital. Two of his three children are Harvard graduates and all three of his children married Harvard graduates. Five of his eight grandchildren have gone to Harvard, as well. Howard loves Harvard, but is frustrated by it as well—frustrated by its innate conservatism and the slow pace of change over time, particularly in its treatment of minorities and women. But he loves that the university draws so many bright people eager to make the world a better place. It was here at Harvard that Howard came into contact with a group of young men and women with whom he has worked on projects to improve the health and well-being of people from inner-city Boston, Africa, Latin America, and beyond.

He was sure he wanted to be a doctor, had really always wanted to be a doctor, and yet as an undergraduate he chose to major in English. The libraries where he went to read Henry James were his home away from the dorm and classrooms; where he worked his way through the details of biology, chemistry, and physics, all in preparation for medical school. In truth, he had little enthusiasm for any of those subjects and tended to learn them in rote fashion. He took the work seriously and was diligent in doing all assigned reading and attending all classes. This was a time when large numbers of legacy students from influential establishment families—wealthy traditionalists from the elite prep schools of the day—spent many hours in the private clubs adjacent to campus and felt no pressure to perform at the highest level academically. This was a time when these young men gathered during school vacations at Pout's Neck, the Hamptons, Hobe Sound, and Palm Beach. Howard, during vacations, repaired to Worcester and toil in Uncle Sidney's shoe store. Howard was of course aware of the sharp class difference between himself and the boys from Exeter, Groton, and St. Paul's as he was aware that many of these students spent considerable hours at the private campus clubs. Howard had little curiosity about this social caste system. (In a 1958 article about the Harvard final clubs in the *Crimson*, Kenneth Auchincloss wrote that "the Clubs generally draw the men of so-called 'good family' and upbringing, and though they are not bound by restrictive codes, only the most exceptional Jew or Negro would have a chance of being accepted."[3] There was a sense of urgency to Howard's work for a couple of reasons. He was well aware that his time as an undergraduate would likely be cut short as a result of the accelerated pace of moving promising undergraduates into medical school to provide doctors for the war effort. And even as he diligently worked his way through his medical school prerequisites, he invested significant time wading into the traditions of great literature. This unusual combination—majoring in English while headed to medical school—exerted significant pressure on Howard to maximize his classroom and study time and he did just that. This was, after all, Harvard, and the academic demands in science and literature were significant.

He found his intellectual passion in the likes of Shakespeare and Henry James. While this was highly unusual for a student on a premed track, it made perfect sense to Howard. In high school, he had done quite a lot of writing and enjoyed it. He felt a genuine sense of intellectual comfort and excitement wading into thick novels by an array of literary giants.

Howard worked joyfully under the tutelage of Theodore Spencer, a renowned Shakespeare scholar, and chose to write his tutorial paper on the novels of Henry James. This was an early glimpse at the mind of young Howard Hiatt. Rare is the teenager eager to take on the density of James's writing and the enormity of his intellect (rarer still the teenaged *medical student* eager to take on James), but Howard plunged in, challenged by the work, exhilarated by the depth and complexity of James's thinking.

World War II changed everything, including Harvard. The urgent need for physicians resulted in Howard applying to medical school after he had been an undergraduate for less than a year, curtailing somewhat his romance with the reading and writing required of an English major. In January 1944, after eleven months as an undergraduate, Howard was admitted to the Harvard Medical School class of 1948 under a program where the army would cover his tuition in return for his service as a military physician. As a medical school student, he would hold the rank of private then receive a promotion to first lieutenant upon graduation.

The anti-Semitism that initially held Howard out of Harvard was present in the medical school application process as well. Howard considered it common knowledge at the time that Jewish students would comprise no more than 10 percent of a medical school class. The culture of Harvard Medical School, like the college, was centered upon elite WASP families. At an introductory medical school dinner with a number of his classmates, the medical school dean of admissions noted with pride the presence in the class of the sons of prominent physicians from well-known medical centers. The dean turned to Howard and said he had forgotten the occupation of Howard's father. Though his dad had spent most of his work life in the United States in the shoe business, Howard mentioned his father's original job upon arriving in the United States from Lithuania. He told the dean that his father was a coal miner. The dean responded smoothly that, of course, excessive inbreeding was undesirable. Howard brushed aside the subtle and not-so-subtle anti-Semitic slights, following his mother's counsel from grade school: *"Well, just ignore him."*

In medical school, Howard continued his sustained academic rigor, devoting most of his waking hours to studying. He considered himself a "grind." Medical school classes in anatomy and chemistry struck him as no more stimulating than his undergraduate science classes. He would still rather immerse himself in Henry James than biology, but, in medical school, that luxury was lost to him.

More interesting to Howard was what he had done just prior to the start of medical school classes when he had undergone two months of basic training at the U.S. Army base in Fort Devens, Massachusetts, about an hour west of Cambridge. Many physicians remain quite comfortably rooted within the strictures of their particular specialty throughout their careers. Many great doctors tend to their discipline—and passion—with attention to little else. Howard was different. From early in high school, he was energized by a deep curiosity—about history, current events, and politics—*about the world*. In high school, he had found real joy in producing and hosting the weekly radio broadcast, "Youth Speaks." His father had influenced him in this area. Al Hiatt read the *Worcester Evening Gazette* each night as well as a weekly Jewish newspaper. He followed the news closely, especially events related to the war, and he was an ardent supporter of President Roosevelt.

At Fort Devens, when he discovered that daily newspapers were unavailable, Howard learned that the NCO's office had access to the Associated Press news wire. With the NCO's approval, Howard reviewed and edited wire copy and broadcast a brief news digest of sorts over the public address system each morning. Most of the news, of course, related to the war and much of that buoyed the spirits of the conscripts.

Howard and his medical school classmates had arrived at Fort Devens in June 1944, soon after the D Day invasion. It was a thrilling time in the United States for it became clear that the epic invasion on the beaches of Normandy had turned the tide of the war. The Allies, it became clear, were destined to win. It was while Howard was at Fort Devens that he learned that the army had a sufficient number of physicians and no longer foresaw an inexhaustible need for new doctors. Thus, Howard and his classmates would be discharged from the service and would return to medical school as civilians, paying their own way. This was not the hardship it would have been had the switch happened today: medical school tuition was then $500 a year.

As the war ended, Howard along with the rest of the world learned more about the extent of the attempted genocide by the Nazis. This, for Howard and his family, was not only political but also personal. Most of the members of Al Hiatt's immediate family were, as far as he knew, still in Lithuania.

Family was important to the Hiatts. Howard grew up with two younger siblings, Arnold, two years his junior, and Marjorie, seven years younger than Howard. Howard and Arnold were highly competitive with one another and fought so often as young boys that their father arrived home one evening with boxing gloves and told the boys to work out their differences in the basement. Howard at the time was chubby while Arnold was slight and their terms of endearment for one another were "Fatso" and "Skinny Runt." Arnold Hiatt recalls that as the oldest child and a spectacularly successful student, Howard was given "a certain kind of pass or grace." He was special and treated as such by their father. Apart from boyhood conflicts between Howard and Arnold, life in the Hiatt household was generally tranquil, although Arnold recalls some tension around his father's constant demands on their mother. "Our father was autocratic," recalls Arnold.

"He was Eastern European and believed women were subordinate. He would tell a story about his own father coming home and having his wife remove his boots. My mother was born in the United States, but my father expected her to cook the dishes he grew up with in Lithuania. She spent a good deal of her time in the kitchen." As a teenager, Arnold Hiatt voiced objections to how his father treated his wife, which angered the father. That conflict, between Arnold and his father, was an ongoing undercurrent in their relationship for many years.

Howard recalls his early relationship with his father as "somewhat distant," but when he got to Harvard it shifted. "A Harvard man" had always been, for Al, the apex, the top of the ladder, and by the time Howard became a doctor—a Harvard doctor to boot—he sensed that his father was respectful and even a bit intimidated by him. He recalls a vivid domestic scene in which he rose up to intervene when his father was verbally abusing his mother and told him that he never wanted to hear him speak that way to her again. "Or else" was the unspoken end of the sentence. Howard never heard his father disrespect his mother again, and his mother later told him that his intervention had made a difference.

Al Hiatt cared very much about his family and would do whatever was in his power to help them. He had sought from his earliest days in this country to bring his parents and his eight siblings to the United States. Two of his older brothers, Nathan and Sidney, did in fact make the journey to the United

States fairly early, and his younger brother, Jacob, a lawyer and a judge, arrived toward the end of the 1930s. Jack, as he was known in the United States, settled in Worcester, living initially with Al's family (and sharing a room with Howard, whom he prepared for his bar mitzvah). Al Hiatt's generosity led to his purchasing a small box-manufacturing company for Jack, which he built into a fabulously successful diversified business which—under his son-in-law—later included among its many properties, the New England Patriots.

Victory in Europe Day came on May 8, 1945. World War II in Europe was finally over. The news was received ecstatically in the United States and, of course, in the Hiatt household as well, but for the Hiatts and other Jewish families, terrible questions remained unanswered. On May 29, Al Hiatt's youngest sibling, Goldie wrote to the family.

My dear ones:

It's been a few days since I returned to Kovno [near the village of Obeliai where the family had lived]. My hope was that I would find Yisroel and the family—but they too were sacrificed to Hitler's murderous actions. And now the loneliness is so great. Most of the Jews of Kovno were eliminated. There are now 500 Jews in Kovno left, and to our tragedy the murderers have taken all that the Jews owned and now they are living and laughing. Now I believe that man is stronger than iron to suffer so much "tsoris" in losing everything and everybody and I have to go on living. I often ask myself the question "Why did I survive?"—I must start to live all over again in loneliness. My only hope is to see you my dear ones, and to tell you how horrible to see all our dear ones obliterated. Beside you, I have no one. In the Jewish group in Kovno, I found your inquiry about me. I have wired you. Now, for the present, I have no place to stay, and now I have to start working.

Christians are living in Yisroel's house now. I was there yesterday and you can imagine how I felt in my heart. It's a wonder my heart didn't burst. Yisroel and his family perished in the ghetto. They were all burned alive during the liquidation. They all perished. 5,000 Jews who were hidden there were burned alive. I was sent to a concentration camp in Germany on March 22, 1945. I was rescued by the Russians. My dear ones, I haven't heard from you for 4 years. Are you all well? Please write often because it takes a long time to receive a letter. Write to the Jewish group in Kovno. I have not as yet got a place to stay and I have no address. I must start working immediately because I can't exist and I have nothing except what I am wearing. That is not important if I could find a member of the family—but they have all perished. The ghetto was demolished on August 14, 1944. Please answer soon.

Your only surviving sister
Goldie

In the final days of the war Goldie had escaped from Auschwitz, where her husband and daughter had been killed. It was Al Hiatt who arranged for her to come to Worcester, together with the husband she had married in the DP camp and their infant son, and it was Al Hiatt who supported them as they became Americans. Howard and his family would learn from Goldie that the family-owned hardware store had been confiscated by a former employee, who had, in a second act of brutality, seized the Chaitowiczes' family home and taken up residence there. Their parents and the other siblings had all been murdered by local people.

What kind of world was this? What was a young medical student—barely twenty years old!—to make of all that surrounded him in the world? He was a Jewish man in a world that had repeatedly sent signals indicating that Jews were to be shunned, marginalized, even killed. But like countless other talented young Jewish men and women at that time, he was undeterred. It was not that he was following his mother's advice to ignore it, surely not. Rather, it only added to an already powerful ambition to do something with his life; to apply the powerful intellect that he knew he possessed to do something that mattered—for himself and his family, and perhaps for others as well.

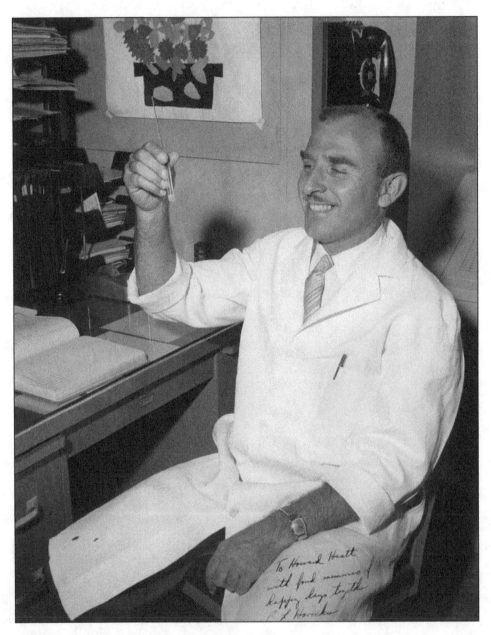

To Howard Heath
with fond memories
happy days together
B. L. Horecker

Figure 2.1
Bernie Horecker, Howard's mentor at NIH and beyond.

2 The Makings of a Physician Scientist

Originally, Howard's ambition throughout medical school was to complete his training and then find his way back to Worcester and set up shop in the general practice of medicine. He felt a deep sense of kinship with Worcester. True, it had none of the worldliness of Cambridge and the Harvard milieu, with its bright students, world-renowned faculty, and faculty rich with Nobel laureates. But Worcester was home and Howard felt comfortable there. His parents were there as were many aunts, uncles, cousins, and friends.

When he completed medical school and embarked upon his residency at Beth Israel Hospital in Boston, he was thrilled to be a real doctor; to have the knowledge and skills to alleviate suffering in other human beings. "I was exhilarated by the realization that, confronted by people who were suffering, I now knew how to help them. And if I didn't, I had more experienced heads available who could advise and guide me to do the best for them."

Howard applied to Massachusetts General Hospital for residency, but he was turned down. His second choice was Beth Israel Hospital where he had done clinical work during medical school. He liked that the hospital was affiliated with Harvard Medical School, though the truth at the time was that it enjoyed a good deal less prestige than Mass General. Nonetheless, Howard was quite happy to begin his residency at Beth Israel in July 1948. He was twenty-three years old and, that summer, had married Doris Bieringer, a beautiful young student at Wellesley College whom Howard had been courting. In Howard's third year of medical school he had met Doris, a Wellesley College senior. A year later, six months after her graduation from college and six months before his graduation from medical school, they were married. That was surely the most important undertaking of his life, because in every important subsequent decision he made—with respect to both personal and career activities—her judgment and advice were crucial. As an added bonus, just a year after they wed, there was a baby on the way.

It is impossible to overstate the important role that Doris came to play in Howard's life. In his memoir he wrote:

> About few things in my life have I ever been more sure. It would be difficult to project what my life would have been like without Doris. She was without question the most supportive person I ever knew. She was extraordinarily insightful—the decisions that I made with respect to my own career were far sounder than they would have been had they not been discussed at length with her. She provided a constant model, close at hand, of deep commitment to and sympathy with (not necessarily the same thing) the problems of under-served and unfortunate people. An almost trivial example: she rarely if ever passed a certain man who asked for help on a street near our home in Cambridge without giving him both some money and a warm greeting. When I walk by this man, I too give him something, but the gesture is not to my credit. I am conscious that I am emulating Doris.
>
> Beyond all else, Doris put aside her own wishes and aspirations to support and promote my career. I wince when I think of the number of times that she gave up something she wanted to do because she felt it might interfere with my plans. In the days when we had but one car, she would often come pick me up at the end of the day to have dinner with our children. I thought little of keeping her waiting outside my office for fifteen or twenty minutes or, I hate to say it, even longer. When she would raise a question about a particularly lengthy delay, I had only to mention a patient suddenly in need of my attention or a medical student who had shown up with a problem that couldn't wait and she would either accept this without question or, rarely, shake her head very slightly and then go on to something else.
>
> It was almost routine for me to return to my lab or my office after dinner while she cleaned up and put the children to bed. When I watch my sons and daughter with their spouses and realize how evenly their chores are divided, I am embarrassed at what Doris accepted as normal. It is true, of course, that the culture has changed considerably, but it seems to me now that my behavior was extreme in its assumption that I was the important partner in the marriage.

In the course of his residency training, Howard broadened his exposure to a subject that had engaged him during medical school. There was a particular class, taught by the legendary Dr. Fuller Albright, that focused on the body's endocrine system. Howard was fascinated by endocrinology and its study of a variety of glandular-related conditions ranging from diabetes to hypertension, osteoporosis to certain cancers. Part of the attraction was Dr. Albright's caring manner. "He captivated students and was known to attract more students than just about any other member of the faculty," recalls Howard. This was fairly remarkable stuff and later, as a resident, Howard had an opportunity to dig more deeply into endocrinology and he found he liked it very much indeed.

Once he made the decision to pursue further work in endocrinology, things moved quickly and triggered a series of events that would take him in just a matter of a few years to New York and Washington, where he would conduct substantive research in his new field. Howard was fortunate to encounter a number of exceptional faculty members whose depth of knowledge and humanity enabled them to distinguish themselves as teachers. Among them was Dr. Hermann Blumgart, who made a point of being available to young doctors seeking help, and so it was that Howard sought him out to ask whether it might make sense for Howard to focus on endocrinology. Without hesitation, Blumgart told Howard that outstanding work was being led at New York Hospital by Dr. Ephraim Shorr, chief of endocrinology at New York Hospital-Cornell Medical School. Based upon Blumgart's recommendation, Howard secured a two-year fellowship in endocrinology. He and Doris moved to New York on July 1, 1950.

There are many scientists whose love of research and discovery is innate. They discover the thrill of the scientific method at an early age, often in high school or even earlier. Certainly, by college many scientists find themselves immersed in the search for some new truth or gathering knowledge in a particularly complex field. Howard was different. Most of his science classes in college and medical school were requirements that he worked his way through in a grinding, mostly joyless fashion. But that all changed when Fuller Albright had engaged him in medical school and it changed again when he entered the research laboratories at New York Hospital. At Beth Israel in Boston there were patients with various endocrine-related conditions, of course, but at New York Hospital, known for its endocrinology service, there were many more patients presenting with a variety of maladies. There were many patients with diseases of the thyroid and the adrenal glands (including Senator John F. Kennedy of Massachusetts who was treated at New York Hospital in the 1950s for his adrenal disease). When not treating patients, Howard worked in the lab, where he was surrounded by an air of vibrant intelligence, even a sense of adventure that he had never before experienced. The other researchers were studying all manner of endocrine-related issues, including thyroid diseases, metabolic disorders, and diseases of the ovaries and testes.

Howard's initial project carried little scientific import, but it was an important moment in his development as a physician/scientist. "I measured the intake of calcium and strontium in rodents' diet and the excretion of those minerals in their urine and feces," he wrote in his memoir. "In retrospect, it was not a particularly valuable exposure to scientific research, but for me at the time it was a beginning" of a way of thinking that would guide him throughout his career; a view of medicine and public health that would guide him in reshaping departments within hospitals as well as an entire graduate school.

While his work in New York was not path-breaking, it was substantial, and Howard's diligence and intelligence were recognized by a number of senior researchers who, in turn, recommended him to colleagues at the National Institutes of Health (NIH) and the Mayo Clinic. On the strength of those recommendations he was invited to join a team going to a newly constructed endocrine unit at NIH in Bethesda, Maryland. Fate, however, intervened. Construction of the new unit fell behind schedule and Howard found himself temporarily without a job. Many decades later, he reflected upon this period during an interview with a writer for the *Boston Globe*, noting that early in his career he

> had an opportunity to go to the National Institutes of Health in Bethesda. When I arrived, the hospital where I was going to work was not quite finished. There was a strike going on. So not wanting to be idle, I found my way into the laboratory of a scientist, a biochemist, who really proved to be extremely important to me. I had never heard of what he was doing and would never have gotten into his lab had there not been this strike. But when I went into his lab, he opened my eyes to what science meant, what it could be. For me, that was, in retrospect, probably one of the most important things that ever happened to me. It did two things for me. It really made me aware of areas that I had no appreciation for, but it also made me aware of how important it was to find a mentor.

The mentor was the avuncular Dr. Bernard Horecker, a well-respected scientist, who took the time to show Howard the way things worked in an advanced scientific research laboratory. Howard was struck by how much more advanced the work was here than what he had been doing back at New York Hospital. "I didn't realize how weak it really was at New York," he recalls. He was essentially feeding various diets to rats and then determining what happened to them. In doing this work, Howard was following the path of a Swedish researcher who was looking into the results of certain nutrition options in rats "and pretty soon I learned that the Swedish scientist I was following had discovered that some of the calculations he had done were mistaken and he discontinued the work." This was a crucial moment, for the reality was that Howard was surrounded in Horecker's lab by sophisticated scientists doing meaningful work. In the center of this was Horecker who, althoughs demanding in his research standards, was also a kind and gentle man. Horecker offered Howard a role in working with him on a project focused on an important enzyme, and overnight Howard was part of the Horecker team. Bernie Horecker took a real interest in the lives and well-being of all the members of the research team. He was demanding, yes, but patient, and always constructive in his guidance to young scientists. This kindness from Horecker, would prove to have a lifelong impact on Howard and his commitment to serve as a mentor to countless young medical students and doctors. (Fifty years after Horecker welcomed Howard into his lab, Howard was visiting the medical program at the University of California at San Francisco and Dr. Robert Wachter, the chief of medicine, introduced him as someone "who has mentored more people than anyone else I know.")

Horecker would go on to become president of the American Society for Biochemistry and Molecular Biology. At the time, he was working to purify the enzyme transketolase, an important part of the process by which cells produce a form of sugar (ribose). This was exciting work with implications for diabetes and other diseases, for it went directly to the essential metabolic process for converting glucose to ribose. An important part of Howard's experience in Horecker's laboratory was meeting an array of ambitious young scientists, men who would go on to assume leadership roles at Albert Einstein Medical School, Memorial Sloan Kettering Hospital, Cornell, Stanford, and Berkeley. This was fertile scientific ground where deep learning was shared on a daily basis. Each workday over lunch, from noon to 1:00 p.m., one of the scientists would report on an aspect of scientific research. Typically, this involved reading the latest articles in a scientific journal and summarizing it for the group then engaging in discussion. The depth and richness of these discussions was unlike anything Howard had ever experienced. This involved some very able young scientists sitting around sharing their own thinking while also reporting on the published insights and findings of others. Howard flourished in this environment. In addition, his studies of the effects of parathyroid hormone on the human kidney (with colleague David Thompson)—the work he had been recruited to carry out at the NIH—resulted in important findings published in the peer-reviewed *Journal of Clinical Investigation.*

The work Horecker was doing zeroed in on the biochemical series of events by which the body makes ribose, the sugar in ribonucleic acid. Horecker's work led to important breakthroughs, including his success in isolating an enzyme called transketolase. A few months after he started work with Horecker, Howard was assigned to work in the clinical facility treating patients with parathyroid disease. He worked during the day at the clinical center, as planned, and worked at the Horecker lab at night and on the weekends. "In my school courses, science had been presented as a series of lessons to be memorized about questions to which the answers were already known," he observed in his private memoir. "By contrast, Bernie gently guided me to the point where I could participate in the excitement of framing the questions and then searching for answers at the lab bench. He opened my eyes to the beauty of science."

Howard was working happily at the NIH when he received a telephone call from his mentor Hermann Blumgart back at Beth Israel. Blumgart explained that he and other leaders at the hospital had decided to establish a medical oncology unit and they wanted Howard to lead it. On the surface, this seemed an odd choice. After all, Howard had no experience with oncology, one of the most challenging fields in medicine. This was a time, the mid-1950s, when many cancers meant a painful and often rapid decline and death, but the fact that so little was known and understood about cancer made the opportunity all the more exciting. Howard was twenty-nine years old at the time [1954] and like many of his colleagues around that age, his general plan was to acquire scientific expertise that would make him a strong candidate to take on an academic position somewhere. Thus, the opportunity offered by Blumgart was thrilling.

Through friends, Howard got in touch with a leading cancer researcher, Dr. Alfred Gellhorn at Columbia Presbyterian Hospital in New York. Howard told Gellhorn that he would be returning to Boston to set up and run a cancer service and, before doing so, he wanted to gain a deeper understanding about the current nature of cancer research and treatment. Gellhorn invited Howard to come to Columbia and see the work there. Howard wondered how long it would take him to do a crash course in oncology, initially thinking it might be a matter of six months to a year. When he shared this thought, Gellhorn laughed heartily. "No, no," he replied.

"I can share with you all that I know in a day but why don't you come for a week."

There were a few drugs administered to cancer patients but none was particularly effective. There was nitrogen mustard, a poison that destroys cancer cells but unfortunately destroyed healthy cells as well. Some antifolate drugs were successful in keeping leukemia in check, but not over the long term. The main lesson Howard learned during his week at Columbia with was that doctors had few tools with which to treat patients with almost any type of cancer. Back in Boston, Howard sought the counsel of Sidney Farber, who was having some success treating leukemia in children, but even Farber did not have effective treatments for adults at that time.

The state of cancer treatment at the BI when Howard took over was rudimentary, as it was at other major hospitals throughout the country. Most of the care was centered upon surgery and the removal of tumors from the breast, bowel, and stomach. The surgeon doing these operations would then follow the patient afterward for however long they were able to survive. Howard's first step was to upgrade the service from a surgical unit to a medical-surgical unit with Howard as the physician leading the medical aspects of care. He also felt the need to add a robust research aspect to the cancer service. After setting up a lab, he kept in close touch with Bernie Horecker at NIH, and the extent of Horecker's influence became clear when Howard sought to learn more about cancer from his studies in molecular biology. Horecker believed, as did the pioneers in the field, that molecular biology had the potential to unlock some of the most difficult challenges in treating patients with cancer. Molecular biology was not only a new approach to the science of medicine, it was an *addition* to medical science. Traditionally, the medical sciences had been anatomy, chemistry, and physiology. So new was the study of molecular biology that there were prominent scientists who did not yet recognize it as a legitimate area for scientific inquiry, but based on work by Horecker and others—including teams of researchers at the Pasteur Institute in Paris—attitudes were changing.

It was becoming clear that at the core of molecular biology lay DNA and RNA, the essential elements of life. It was closely tied to chemistry and biology, but it added a new dimension. It drew scientists into a deeper search to understand genetic makeup. A critical question involved the mechanisms through which genes were transcribed into RNA and, in turn, what the mechanism was for morphing RNA into a protein. Howard was enthralled by these questions and by the possibility that additional research could advance basic scientific understanding in important ways. At Beth Israel, he went about recruiting talented people trained in fundamental science. Some were physicians with clinical training, others held PhD degrees and had never worked outside a research laboratory. In the 1950s very few people Howard knew grasped the potential applications of biomedical study on patient care. Howard wanted to change that. With funding from the National Cancer Institute Howard opened his own laboratory and continued the research work he had started under Bernie Horecker. He sought to determine whether the pathway leading to ribose, the sugar component of RNA, was different in cancer cells versus healthy cells. Howard found that the pathway was not different, a finding that was not of great significance, but it was important enough to earn Howard an invitation as one of the presenters to the plenary session of the annual American Society for Clinical Investigation meeting in Atlantic City. This presentation along with the publication of his work brought about numerous invitations for Howard to speak at medical schools and medical meetings around the country, which all served to enhance the standing and reputation of Beth Israel Hospital.

Even though Howard was in Boston and Bernie Horecker was at the NIH, the two men continued their joint research efforts together and coauthored a number of important papers on messenger RNA and related topics. It would be difficult to overstate Horecker's influence on Howard. In 1958, when Howard was thirty-three years old, Horecker suggested that for Howard to pursue his interest in understanding cancer in a much deeper way, he needed to head off to Paris and work with the researchers at the Pasteur Institute. At the time, the most basic question in the field of oncology remained unanswered: *What is the mechanism by which human cells become cancerous?* To try and answer that question—or any aspect of it, Horecker said—you must immerse yourself in this new field of molecular biology. Horecker himself had spent a year at the Pasteur and knew the scientists there well and upon Horecker's recommendation, Howard was invited to join the team for a twelve-month period. When the invitation to the Pasteur came in 1960, Howard had been at the BI for just four years. He had in no way earned the right to any sort of sabbatical, yet when he explained the situation to Blumgart, the older man was nothing but encouraging. *Go,* said Dr. Blumgart, and Howard was off to Paris for a year.

The Pasteur Institute was where the molecular biology revolution took root. There was important work in the field being done at Caltech, and in England at Cambridge University, but scientists working on molecular biology—whether they were from the United States, the UK, Sweden, Denmark, or elsewhere—made a point of finding their way to Paris. The institute was named for the nineteenth-century chemist who proved to be one of the great scientific minds in history. The opportunity to work with the scientists at the Pasteur was both exciting and daunting. These were some of the giants in the world of science, men who would go on to win the Nobel Prize. Howard, by contrast, was a young physician with one foot in the world of scientific research and the other in clinical treatment of patients. Jacques Monod, who led the work in molecular biology at Pasteur, gave Howard a warm welcome upon his arrival in Paris and arranged to have his graduate student, Francois Gros, serve as Howard's mentor. In his memoir, Howard is self-effacing about his humble approach to the work in Paris:

> The first assignment Francois gave me was to repeat an experiment that he, Francois, had carried out recently. I did so and got results that were very different from those that he had gotten on a couple of previous occasions. At one o'clock the following day, Monod, as he did almost every day, sat on a lab bench and went over the results of the day's experiment. When he heard the results that I had obtained, Monod was initially puzzled and then seemed pleased. We all followed him into the adjacent library, where he went to the board and worked my result into a scheme that seemed to cast doubt on the major hypothesis on which the lab was working at that time. He expressed pleasure at this result and said that he hadn't been fully convinced by the evidence to date, and "perhaps Howard is telling us that we have to rethink our present hypothesis."
>
> I did the experiment again, and on this occasion, came up with results that were precisely those that Francois had been getting. I presented them to Monod the following day. Again, the group went to the board in the library, and Jacques expressed great relief that no new theory was required. He made me feel as though I were really a contributor rather than the mistaken source of the doubt.

In reality, Howard was part of the team seeking to answer a central question at that time in the field of molecular biology: *How are instructions contained in the DNA translated into the proteins that carry out the cell's functions?* Scientists had established that information contained within DNA was communicated to proteins, but no one had discovered *how* that happened. The process of transferring the information, says Howard, was a "black box." Scientists knew that the information contained within an individual's DNA was transmitted

to proteins that then determined that someone had blue eyes while someone else would have brown eyes. How was that information transported and
conveyed?

The work was demanding. On numerous occasions experiments required
that Howard work late into the night, but he did not mind, for he loved the
work and the search for answers to such fundamental and potentially path-
breaking questions. He had trained as a physician working with patients, of
course, but he also possessed an ever-growing background in science. There
was something about the Paris work—the eminent scientists with whom he
worked, the possibility of success. It was, he noted in his memoir, the most
exciting scientific exploration he had ever done.

> Almost every day at the lab contained a new and exciting undertaking: another
> question about our hypothesis, another experiment to address that question.
> Virtually all of the experiments involved *Escherichia coli*, bacteria that reproduce
> quickly, as quickly as every twenty minutes. For our experiments, they were placed
> to grow in the presence of minute quantities of a radioactive substance. After
> several generations (a matter of hours, not years), the bacteria were harvested and
> homogenized and their contents analyzed.
>
> In many experiments the analysis involved a sucrose gradient—a procedure
> in which the cell contents are layered in a plastic tube containing a solution of
> sucrose and the tube is then spun at very high speeds for several hours to sepa-
> rate various cell constituents. At the end of that time, the bottom of the tube is
> pierced, and drops are collected, as they come out, in a succession of glass tubes.
> The sucrose gradient separated the constituents according to weight, the lighter
> ones at the top and the denser at the bottom.

This process solved the mystery. It revealed what is known as messenger
RNA,

> the lightest and most ephemeral of the cell constituents, at one level of the tubes
> while the other cell constituents, including the RNA from other parts of the cell,
> were at other levels. We found that no matter how short the period of time in
> which the bacteria were left to reproduce, the mRNA was "labeled," or marked with
> radioactivity, when other constituents were not. This told us it was formed first.
> The order told us that this newly recognized RNA component, mRNA, existed in
> all cells.

As is so often the case with critically important scientific puzzles, a number of researchers on different teams were involved in pursuit of messenger
RNA. While they were competing to find the answer, there was nonetheless a collaborative spirit among the two teams. These were men able to

subjugate their natural instinct for recognition within the scientific community in favor of a collaborative approach that would prove to yield excellent results from both teams. One group was at the Pasteur Institute, of course, led by Jacques Monod and Jacob with Gros and Howard conducting the bulk of the actual experiments within the lab. Also helping from long distance was James Watson at Harvard, who would go on to win the Nobel Prize for his work on the DNA double helix, while Jacob and Monod would win the Nobel prize for their discoveries about messenger RNA. The other group was centered at Caltech, led by Matthew Meselson, and included Sydney Brenner from Cambridge, England, and Francois Jacob, who served on both the Pasteur and Caltech teams. Since Jacob participated on both teams he was able to share new information and discoveries with each group, thus accelerating the overall pace of inquiry. As though to put an exclamation point on this appealing collaborative culture, the Caltech team completed their paper on the work before the Pasteur team completed theirs. The Caltech team surely could have published first, but they chose to wait until the Pasteur group had completed their paper and both were published in *Nature* (May 13, 1961). This reflected an unusual level of collaboration, trust, and respect between the two competing teams, something that would be extremely rare now, if it were to occur at all. In recognition of the importance of Howard's work on the project, he was listed as one of the authors of the paper. The discovery found that a messenger RNA molecule in a cell would travel from the DNA nucleus with its precious cargo of information. The molecule would find its way to the cytoplasm where protein synthesis occurred to deliver the information. During a process known as transcription, the information contained within DNA is transferred into messenger RNA, whose molecules carry the codes of just a single protein.

This was a heady time in Howard's life. He was working in the lab with three scientists who would go on to win Nobel prizes. In 1961 the first International Congress of Biochemistry was held in Moscow and Howard was selected to attend the conference with Francois Jacob. Seeing that Howard was representing Monod and listed as a delegate from France, one American scientist even complimented Howard on his English. ("My mother was American," was Howard's reply.) For a young researcher to travel to the other world superpower at the height of the Cold War and collaborate with scientists from throughout the world was a particularly exciting experience.

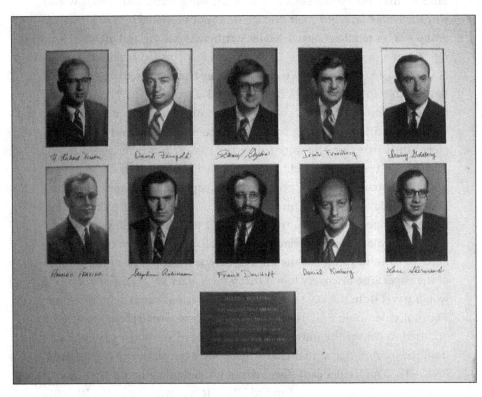

Figure 3.1
Hiatt's Hoplites.

3 Change Agent: Bringing a Science Base to Medicine

Dr. Hermann Blumgart's decision to retire as chief of medicine at Beth Israel may not have been a surprise—he had reached the mandatory retirement age for Harvard Medical School professors of sixty-five—but it was a bit of a shock to people throughout the organization. Blumgart had distinguished himself as quite a remarkable clinician, so much so that in the years to come several prestigious awards from medical societies would be granted in his name. A search committee seeking to identify a worthy successor to Dr. Blumgart, quickly settled upon a physician then serving as chairman of the Department of Medicine at Southwestern Medical School. When the offer from Beth Israel was tendered, however, the folks at Southwestern countered with a generous package and the man chose to remain at Southwestern.

The decision by this doctor to turn down Beth Israel would prove one of the more fortuitous moments of Howard Hiatt's life. The Beth Israel search committee reacted quickly, huddling to discuss alternatives. That evening, as Howard was working in the cold room of his research laboratory, a committee member burst in and excitedly informed Howard that he was the committee's choice to ascend to the position. Howard was thrilled. At one level the decision to accept the new position was quite simple: It was an extraordinary honor and professional opportunity. At the same, time, however, it would mean that Howard's time for research would be seriously curtailed. This was a painful sacrifice, yet it was one he was willing to make. He loved the lab. He loved basic research. There was nothing else quite like probing the essence of cells and their mind-bogglingly efficient and often mysterious functions. Yet he recognized, as he wrote in his private memoir, that "it would be an exciting time to be building a department because of the pace with which biological science was yielding greater understanding of human illness and, as a result, more effective ways of preventing and treating it." And he was convinced that "academic medicine could profit greatly from the application of the 'new biology'" to medical problems. "I recognized that I would be reducing considerably my time in the lab but the opportunity to recruit a substantial number of bright young people in all of the medical fields to conduct research and treat patients in clinic was an opportunity I couldn't turn down. The chance to remake a department of medicine into a modern unit allying new scientific understanding with the management of patients was irresistible," Howard wrote in his memoir.

He recognized that he was in a position with considerable leverage and he sought to use that leverage in a way that would enable him to gather the resources he would need to build a new department—a different kind of medical department. He told the hospital leaders, including the members of the board of trustees, that in order to build a world class department of medicine he would need a significant expansion of laboratory research space, and the hospital's president assured Howard that the next newly constructed building at the hospital would be devoted to the research mission.

As the new chief of medicine Howard received a warm reception from other department heads. This could have been tricky and surely would have been uncomfortable at other medical centers with a less collegial culture. He was but thirty-seven years old, quite young to be selected as chairman of the department of medicine, the most influential of department chiefs at most major medical centers. The other heads of departments—surgery, radiology, pathology, and others—were considerably older, yet they were welcoming and supportive.

It may be simplistic to divide Howard Hiatt's career into two distinct roles, but there is some truth to it. As a younger man, he was a mentee who benefitted from the generous mentoring of older, more experienced men. Then, at a certain point, Howard crossed over from being a mentee to being a mentor, guiding dozens, scores, perhaps hundreds of talented young students and doctors. As he took over at Beth Israel, he was still squarely in the mentee category and one of his first actions as chief was to seek advice from two highly respected chiefs of departments of medicine. Walter Bauer and Robert Loeb, at Massachusetts General Hospital and Columbia-Presbyterian Hospital respectively, served as models for Howard. "They had built the kinds of departments that I wanted to build at Beth Israel," Howard wrote in his memoir. "Both had picked young faculty members trained in clinical medicine for their departments, sent them off to biological science labs for research training and then brought them back to build within their departments units of cardiology, endocrinology, pulmonary, kidney and so forth, informed by laboratory research."

Given the mission, the importance of new laboratory space could not be overstated. As he interviewed and recruited people, he held out the shining promise of a brand new, state-of-the-art research building more modern than anything else in town. His first recruit was Irving Goldberg, MD, PhD, from the University of Chicago Medical School He had been in Loeb's department and Loeb had recommended him, describing him as "the kind of chief resident who let me sleep at night." Goldberg had recently been tenured at Chicago and when Howard wrote to him in 1963 inquiring whether he might consider coming to Beth Israel, Goldberg hesitated. The prospect of working with Howard to build a great faculty was appealing to Goldberg, however, and he agreed to come to Beth Israel, Howard wrote, "on condition that laboratory space to accommodate the work he had in mind would soon be available. I assured him it would."

Irv Goldberg was just the kind of young scientist/clinician Howard wanted to add to the BI department of medicine. "Harvard in those years had a reputation of either bringing in very senior people who were tenured or bringing in junior people who would then have a tough time getting tenure at Harvard," recalls Goldberg, who made it clear to Howard that he would not consider giving up tenure at Chicago and coming to the BI unless he was granted tenure at Harvard Medical School. Howard went to work on this and twisted enough arms to meet Goldberg's requirement. Irv Goldberg, Howard's first major hire to help bring Beth Israel to a world-class level, arrived there in 1964.

The two men hit it off right from the start in part, of course, as a result of their mutual desire to do great work in medicine, but also owing to shared past experiences. Goldberg had graduated at the top of his high school class in Hartford, Connecticut, and his aspiration to attend Yale was dashed when his high school principal told him that "Yale doesn't give scholarships to Jews." Goldberg shifted gears and attended Trinity College, where he commuted to classes near his home in Hartford and then joined the navy during the war. After the war he went to Yale Medical School, which was accepting additional numbers of Connecticut residents to head off an effort by the University of Connecticut to start its own medical school. Goldberg had done his residency at Columbia, under Dr. Robert F. Loeb, worked in a biochemistry lab there for a time, and then was sent by Loeb to Rockefeller University for his PhD. At Rockefeller he had worked under the tutelage of Nobel Laureate Fritz Lippman.

Goldberg went on to play a central role in building the BI Department of Medicine into one with a renowned reputation, but, in an interview years later, he recalls that he almost didn't accept Howard's offer. "I wasn't that interested in going to a Jewish hospital," he recalls, "because that was the only place people like me could go at one point." But he was pleased with the situation at Beth Israel where Howard Hiatt worked "to make sure that the environment was conducive to doing serious biomedical science."

Howard's career in medicine had proceeded along a smooth pathway, one success after another: prestigious jobs, fellowships, working with some of the great scientific minds in the world, publishing in impressive journals about breakthroughs that mattered. But all careers are marked by reversals and one of the measures of people is how they handle those moments. At Beth Israel, the executive and board leadership was clear on Howard's need for new laboratory space. He had received an ironclad promise for that space from Sidney Lee, the hospital CEO, and Howard's expectation was that the space would be constructed by the start of 1966. Six months prior to that date, however, Lee sat down with Howard and broke the bad news: Lee had met with board members and they had changed plans. The next new building would not be for research, but instead would go for patient care. Howard was taken aback. He reminded Lee of the promise he had made. "But we've had a change of mind," Lee explained. "It will be okay. The *next* building will be for research." But Howard had made a promise to Irv Goldberg concerning the research space and that promise had been crucial in attracting Irv from Chicago. And that promise was part of the pitch Howard was making to numerous other, talented physician-researchers. Howard and Sidney Lee went back as the exchange grew increasingly tense. Howard wanted to go to the trustees and explain how urgent it was to him that his promise to Irv be kept; how critically important it was to what he was just starting to build to have the appropriate research space.

Howard explained that he had made promises about a new research facility not only to Goldberg but also to others, including Frank Davidoff, another physician Howard sought to recruit. "I said that I intended to keep my promises," Howard recalled. "He said 'you have my word' that the next building will be a research facility,' and I said, 'I had your word before. You've got to change this decision.' " "Sorry," Lee said. "The decision is final. Let's move on." But Howard had no intention of accepting the decision and moving on. A deal was a deal and Lee had broken his word and now Howard would be breaking his word to Irv Goldberg. He was as angry as he was clear-minded. Principles mattered. Commitments mattered. Keeping your word mattered.

On July 22, 1965, Howard's fortieth birthday, he wrote a letter to Sidney Lee at Beth Israel Hospital, with a copy to George Packer Berry, dean of the Harvard Medical School, resigning his positions at the medical school and the hospital. The next day, he took his family on a long-planned vacation to the southwest.

As Howard and Doris Hiatt traveled through the southwest with their children, Howard found it difficult to get his mind off of the fact that he had given up the Blumgart professorship of medicine at one of the most prestigious medical schools in the world, but he knew he could not work in an environment where foundational commitments were cast aside. He felt certain it was the right thing to do and he was confident that Irv Goldberg, Frank Davidoff, and the others to whom he had made promises would understand his action. He simply could not tolerate a situation where specific promises were made to him and then broken.

Four days into the trip a call came to the hotel from Samuel Slosberg, chairman of the Beth Israel board. He asked Howard to return to Boston the next day to meet with trustees to try and resolve the situation. Reluctantly leaving Doris with three children in a car in Utah, Howard traveled back to Boston and Doris and the children went on to California. At the meeting of trustees, board members said they recognized the significance of what he was doing and they had changed their collective mind. The next building would, in fact, be a research facility and Howard could continue his recruitment efforts with that promise. But this would happen only if Howard withdrew his resignation. He did so. Soon thereafter, the hospital president departed from Beth Israel.

The idea was to recruit the brightest young minds he could find: young men and women with a passion for both clinical medicine and scientific research, who wanted to teach as well, to share their accumulated knowledge and insights with other physicians and medical students. Since completing his training as a doctor, Howard had invested significant time in research and, in so doing, had deepened his understanding of disease. This investment in research also led him to explore and understand a much broader array of treatments for patients than he otherwise would have understood. He wanted intellectually ambitious and curious men and women who were eager to join an adventure where they would care for patients and explore new regions of science. Word quickly circulated throughout the medical community that something special was happening at Beth Israel Hospital and it became a magnet for smart young men and women who wanted to be great doctors, yes, but aspired also to conduct research and teach.

Pleased with his successful recruitment of Irv Goldberg and the resolution of the research building issue, Howard sought to attract doctors from Massachusetts General Hospital, from Columbia-Presbyterian in New York, from the NIH, and from the University of Wisconsin at Madison, where Dr. Warner Slack was doing work that Howard admired involving computers and their application in medicine. Howard learned of Slack's work through Dr. Howard Bleich, a physician within Howard's department at Beth Israel. Bleich spoke with great enthusiasm about the thinking Slack and his colleagues were doing in Madison. Howard learned that Slack had created in 1965 a program that allowed a patient to give a medical history to a computer— the first that that had ever been done. The result was one of the first articles published in the *New England Journal of Medicine* concerning computers in medicine.

The article caught Howard's attention. It was intelligent and well presented and Howard wanted to know more—about Slack and about the potential of computers in medicine. Howard was in the room for a presentation Slack gave at Beth Israel in 1969 and Howard came away from that event thinking that Slack was just the kind of smart, innovative young doctor he wanted within the Department of Medicine. He spoke with Dr. Bleich, who suggested that perhaps Howard should consider asking Slack to join the staff at Beth Israel. Howard met with Slack a couple of times in late 1969 and early 1970 and asked whether he might consider coming to the BI to create a Division of Clinical Computing within the Department of Medicine in partnership with Howard Bleich. The purpose of the division would be to explore ways computers might be harnessed to help physicians provide better care for patients. Slack was very happy at Wisconsin, but the offer was too good to decline and in the fall of 1970 he joined the team at the BI.

"Howard had a way of supporting our work and making us feel appreciated," recalls Slack. "I was at Beth Israel for two years before Howard left to become dean of the school of public health but those two years I grew to revere him." Slack and Bleich developed one of the first hospital-wide computer systems, enabling doctors to receive a variety of clinical information more quickly than before. Slack and Bleich were later asked to build a similar system at Brigham and Women's Hospital.

Around the same time, at the University of Washington School of Medicine in Seattle, Tony Komaroff was hanging out during summer break with two friends who were students at Harvard Medical School. When Tony told them his plan was to do a fellowship at Boston City Hospital, his friends both urged him to go to Beth Israel instead. When he asked why, the two friends said simultaneously: "Howard Hiatt!" Tony followed his friends' advice, applied to the BI and was accepted.

"Howard was a very young chairman of the department of medicine and my friends told me that he was transforming the place and when I got there I could see what they were talking about" recalls Komaroff. "It was my first experience with how profoundly a leader can affect an institution. Beth Israel was a traditional, excellent hospital with some eminent faculty members, but when Howard was appointed chairman of medicine it rapidly became the hot place for medical students, medical residents, and young faculty. It was a time of genuine excitement, an aura about the place that wasn't there at the other more famous hospitals, Mass General and the Brigham."

No single characteristic drew people to Howard. Rather, says Komaroff, it was a combination things, including the fact that he was unusually young to be a department chair at a time when a youth culture in the United States was blossoming. Howard also possessed an unusually powerful intellect. Komaroff recalls that "in a world of *very* smart people he was extraordinarily smart. He was brilliant *and* he was charismatic. Everyone wanted to know what he thought and to engage with him in some way. All of the younger students, residents, and fellows felt like they were one of his mentees and that he had their best interest in his mind. You don't often feel that way about your leader."

Finally, he was a serious scientist. "This was the time of the birth of the molecular biology revolution and Howard was one of the few academics in Boston rooted in molecular biology. He had worked with the best people in the world, with the team at Pasteur and with Jim Watson. And there was a sense that molecular biology would be the future of laboratory medical science."

It said something important about Howard that he did not chose to have his medical team focus on molecular biology to the exclusion of other pursuits. He surely could have done so and there is a case to be made for his having done so, yet he recognized that the bright young people coming to the BI had diverse interests and he knew from experience that pursuing one's medical and scientific passion was essential to productivity and happiness in the intense world of a tertiary care hospital. "He wanted all his trainees to work on problems that were really important," says Komaroff. "His breadth of vision was unusual for what he defined as important. It was a small department and he could have focused all of his energy on building a department infused with molecular biology with the goal of changing medicine. And molecular biology was an extremely important part of what was happening at the hospital then, but Howard also cared deeply about and wanted to emphasize other things."

He also saw—and in this sense he was a couple of decades ahead of the best thinking in healthcare—that medical resources in the United States were used inefficiently. He was one of the early thinkers who recognized that expensive and in some cases harmful tests were being given to people without much of an evidence base to indicate that the tests were effective.

"Before anyone else was talking about these issues that are now commonplace Howard was thinking carefully about them and raising questions about benefits of medical tests and interventions versus risks and asking about benefits versus expense—the cost of these interventions," says Komaroff. "Howard was very interested in the failings of American medicine in the sense that medical care was poorly distributed in the wealthiest society in the history of creation. That was a passion for him."

Many years later, Komaroff authored an article that was part of a JAMA series entitled "Scientific Discovery and the Future of Medicine," in which he wrote: "Why should the accomplishments of modern biology matter to practicing physicians and their patients? Perhaps the answer is obvious, but when a physician is in the midst of a busy day in practice, it can be hard to care. It is difficult enough to keep up with new knowledge that immediately affects practice. It is even more difficult to keep up with and appreciate advances in modern biology that may affect practice in the future. The series helps in appreciating what is happening." As part of the series, Komaroff wrote about the "birth of modern biological research":

It is hardly an exaggeration to say that "modern biology" is one of the great intellectual accomplishments in human history. The birth of modern biology (notably molecular biology) occurred in 1944 when 3 physicians—Oswald Avery, Colin MacLeod, and Maclyn McCarty—reported that a "transforming substance" from dead virulent pneumococci could permanently transfer virulence to living nonvirulent pneumococci. Avery likened that "transforming substance" to a gene, because it appeared to have the 2 properties required of a gene: it could copy itself, and it could transform the structure and function of the cell through directing the production of particular proteins. The meticulous experiments by Avery strongly argued that the transforming substance was DNA.

Spurred by Avery's results, a decade later James Watson and Francis Crick deduced the molecular structure of DNA. That structure immediately suggested how a gene could copy itself. After a decade more of work, it also became clear how genes direct the production of specific proteins. These fundamental discoveries transformed both biology and medicine over the past half century.

The most apparent measure of the value of modern biology is the array of tools it has provided to prevent or cure disease. Certain biotechnologies (some linked to computing technologies) have profoundly improved understanding the pathogenesis of diseases, leading to remarkable improvements in diagnosis and treatment.

Komaroff notes that Howard was working at the Pasteur Institute at a crucial moment in the modern history of biological science and that messenger RNA was a key discovery. "Howard was there at the birth of molecular biology," he says.

One of the most unusual recruits during Howard's time as chief was Herb Sherman, an MIT-trained engineer with no medical background. In his memoir, Howard referred to Sherman as "a glorious anomaly" whose "presence at the BI was an early and vivid example of the enormous benefits of cross-fertilization, the result of looking at the practices of one profession with the training of another." Sherman worked at the MIT Lincoln Laboratory, an elite research and development division within MIT devoted to national defense and funded by the United States government. The roots of Lincoln Laboratory grew out of the MIT department of physics, where scientists developed advanced radar systems that played an essential role in winning World War II.

Like his predecessors at Lincoln, Sherman was focused on a national defense project involving a communications satellite. He had no particular interest in medicine, until, that is, his wife fell ill and required advanced cardiac surgery to replace a valve. When Herb and Howard met, quite by

chance at a cocktail party, Sherman explained to Howard that he was aston-
ished by what he discovered when he did some research into the use of a
porcine valve such as the one implanted in his wife. Sherman asked Howard: "Did you know that there was only one experiment in the literature on
the effectiveness of using pig valves, and that experiment was with twelve
dogs? If I put up a satellite with so little experimental research behind it, I
would lose my job."

Howard was drawn to Sherman's inquisitive mind, the way Sherman
thought differently about medicine than most people. He liked that Sherman brought the perspective of science without medicine. It was a clean slate
in a way that allowed Sherman to question everything, which is precisely
what he did. For many physicians, perhaps particularly a chief of department,
this might have been distracting or even annoying. Howard embraced it,
recalling in his memoir that "Sherman cared about what worked and what
didn't. He brought no philosophical biases to his inquiries, had no a priori
theories. He would just ask, 'Does this seem to make sense?' Did it make
sense to put pigs' valves in humans on the strength of one experiment? If it
didn't make sense to him, he would start to think of ways in which things
could be changed so that it did."

As much as Howard was drawn to Sherman and his way of approach-
ing problems, Sherman was attracted to Howard and the medical field. His
wife's surgery had sent Sherman off on a research mission to try and understand how medical decisions were made. This interest got him talking with
colleagues at Lincoln Laboratory and Sherman approached Howard with
an idea: Would Howard be interested in having Sherman and a Lincoln
colleague work with Howard and his team with an eye toward a possible
affiliation between Beth Israel Hospital and Lincoln Laboratory? Howard
loved the idea.

The level of interest on the part of Lincoln Lab became clear when Sherman and another colleague from Lincoln, engineer Barney Reiffen, were
granted a paid leave of absence to work at Beth Israel. Howard was the ben-
eficiary of two superb engineering minds at no cost! It was a remarkable gift.
After spending some time observing, Sherman said to Howard:

> Medicine is different. If someone came into my office looking for an engineer and
> told me, "I want to build a bridge like the one in Brooklyn," the first thing I'd do
> is get down a book by somebody who had built such a bridge, and I'd say, "Here

is how they did it, let's go." But if I went into a doctor's office and said, "I have a pain in my belly," and the doctor went to a book on the shelf behind him to look up pain in the belly, I'd say that's not a doctor I'd want to go to.

The year was 1968, but Sherman's thinking was more in line with trends four decades later when the concept of having all members of the team work to the top of their license—practicing to the full extent of their education and training—became something most organizations adopted, at least in theory. Sherman asked Howard "whether people with less training could perform some key tasks that were necessary but, not requiring much skill, perhaps a little boring and maybe even annoying to busy doctors," Howard wrote in his memoir:

> Wouldn't it be more efficient to have some of these tasks performed by non-physicians? They might not only save the doctors time but also perform these functions better because they would be focusing on them alone. And, Sherman and Reiffen observed, doctors didn't always do them very well. For example, diabetic patients need their feet examined to be sure they are not developing sores they are unaware of that can become infected and lead to gangrene. After discussions with Sherman and Barney, the doctors in the diabetes clinic assigned that task at the BI to nurses and nurses' aides. Our follow-up studies showed that reassigning this task did save doctors'time, of course, but more important, it also appeared to have improved patient care.

Sherman saw the messiness of medicine. As an engineer, the idea of standardization made sense to Sherman. If there was a best way to do something in engineering engineers followed that path. Not so in medicine he saw. There was little effort to identify the best practice and no effort—at least none discernible to Sherman—to standardize best practices. In 2016, standardization in many aspects of medicine is widely recognized as contributing to better outcomes and financial efficiency. Howard wrote in his memoir:

> Sherman noticed that doctors approached patients with the same presenting complaint in very different ways. There seemed to be no consistency as to what was done when a patient walked in and said, for example, "My throat is sore." Some doctors reached for a tongue suppressor, some took the patient's temperature, some interviewed the patient at length. Sherman asked whether there wasn't a "right" way to do things, in line with the current level of medical knowledge. Was there an order in which questions should be asked and examinations should be undertaken, and if there was, shouldn't we have some sort of system that says everyone who cares for a patient with a sore throat should do these things in this order on the initial examination?

The scientist in Howard found the presence of Sherman quite thrilling. Howard was not certain what sort of advances might come of Sherman's presence and his application of engineering techniques and principles to medicine, but he felt a sense of anticipation that some important ground could be broken.

Sherman and Reiffen were joined in their efforts by Dr. Tony Komaroff, who had come to the Beth Israel Hospital as a medical resident and today is a distinguished professor of medicine at Harvard Medical School. They were working on an issue that had both surprised and puzzled Sherman as he had seen his wife go through her medical challenges. The issue involved how doctors make decisions. Sherman was taken aback by what he considered individualistic approaches by physicians in decision-making. This approach, while typically based on extensive education and training, was nothing more than haphazard when seen through an engineering lens. Sherman and other engineers had applied algorithms in their decision-making process and, by doing so, brought mathematical consistency to the process. Not so in medicine, at least not as far as Sherman was able to determine.

"Howard saw that molecular biology would play an important role in medicine going forward and he also saw, before most others, that information technology would play an important role as well," says Komaroff. "In the mid-seventies computer technology had virtually no place yet in the practice of medicine anywhere in the world and Howard said something should be done. He didn't know what should be done but he didn't care about that. He knew that the way to approach the issue was to bring in Sherman and his team and let them observe and study and then listen to them. He instinctively believed that with powerful new computing technology that somehow in medicine we would be able to make more rational decisions."

It was an opportune time to explore the possibilities inherent in technology. Throughout medicine in the 1960s was a commonly held belief that the country was experiencing a shortage of physicians and that the problem was likely to grow more acute. The question was whether steps could be taken to change the work doctors did—to shift some work typically done by physicians to other members of the healthcare team. There were any number of tasks physicians were doing routinely that surely did not require a medical school education to do. The issue was to identify these things and figure out who else on the care delivery team would be able to do these things reliably.

Howard formed a hybrid team of physicians and computer scientists, and called it the Ambulatory Care Project, a joint venture between Beth Israel and MIT's Lincoln Lab. A senior physician leader had been appointed but left Beth Israel not long after. Howard then appointed Komaroff as the medical director of the Ambulatory Care Project at the tender age of just thirty. Komaroff was thrilled yet somewhat daunted by the prospect of taking on such a role barely a year out of his residency, but Howard provided full support and Komaroff got to work directly with Sherman and Reiffen and other members of the MIT team, most of whom had moved their work space over to the BI.

Howard had blessed a program where engineers from MIT who had worked on rockets and radar were charged with altering the care delivery process in medicine. This work was, by definition, disruptive. More traditional medical school faculty members could be forgiven for viewing this with a degree of suspicion.

Komaroff was thrilled working with Sherman, Reiffen and their colleagues. "We were thinking that computers would help guide health care professionals in their decision-making," he says. "Specifically, we thought that computer algorithms could individualize care for patients with generally the same problem. Algorithms would explicitly specify what questions should be asked, what parts of the physical examination should be done, and what tests ordered—for example, in patients with diabetes coming for a checkup. The algorithms would specify things that needed to be done in every diabetic patient, regardless, and other things that needed to be done only in some patients based on their answers to questions, or the results of their physical examination. At first, we assumed that such algorithms would be so complicated you would have to use a computer to present them."

It did not take long before the team working on this project acknowledged that if they were to construct the world's greatest computer-based algorithm, nobody would use it owing to the prohibitive computer cost. This acknowledgment added to the challenge before the team. Challenge number one was to design the algorithms for a variety of practices and procedures that would enable minimally trained nonphysicians to perform highly useful clinical tasks. Challenge number two was to see if the algorithm could be represented on paper so that caregivers in the clinic would be able to be guided by algorithms clamped on a clipboard. In other words, these MIT computer geeks had to come up with a way of representing complex medical logic that would involve *not* using computers.

Sherman, Reiffen, Tony Komaroff, and the other team members embraced the twin challenges and developed techniques for representing the complex medical logic on one side of a sheet of paper.

The next decision was to identify the type of non-physician to use the algorithms. The first thought was nurses. But Komaroff knew—and Sherman could see—that nurses were already working at full capacity. Moreover, they wondered if it required the extensive education received by nurses to function in such a role.

"We thought you can teach smart people without a college education how to do the ten things every diabetic patient coming for a return visit needs to have done before seeing the doctor," says Komaroff. "We focused on briefly-trained physician assistants, often people aspiring to become fully-trained physician assistants and created a step in the process prior to the doctor seeing the patient where the physician's assistant would ask a series of questions based on the algorithms that we had developed."

The question was whether a person with a high-school education could deliver reliable, high-quality care to every patient every time at a lower cost than what a doctor would charge. This was an important element. Howard was clear in his desire that the teams explore ways to reduce the financial waste in healthcare delivery. He believed excessive spending in healthcare was depriving other important social needs of funding and he took seriously a responsibility in medicine to spend money wisely, without waste.

Going into the experiments, Tony Komaroff had a theory: that the high-school educated people Sherman and the teams would train might actually do a *better* job than doctors in the part of the exam of diabetes patients assigned to them. How remarkable that would be! In part, his belief was based on the knowledge that even though doctors knew they were supposed to examine the feet of patients with diabetes, for example, physicians pressed for time did not always do so. This was dangerous. Diabetic patients could develop sores on their feet and, as a result of nerve damage, they would be unaware the sores were there. These sores were prone to infection if untreated and in some cases patients with diabetes had to have an infected foot amputated.

The physicians' assistants were well trained and when Tony and the others observed their work they saw that the physicians' assistants went through the paper form with a religious commitment to do all of the work the algorithm prescribed. The result of this experiment was enlightening.

"We demonstrated that people with no more than a high school education could deliver high quality, less expensive care," says Komaroff. "By several measures of medical outcomes the patients did *better* than when physicians alone did that work because the doctors were so pressed for time that although they knew it was important, for example, to check the feet of diabetic patients the fact was that they often did not do so. With the new team, the patient's feet were examined every time just as everything else on the checklist was asked or examined every time. We found that with the medical assistants doing this work patients were being more thoroughly evaluated and doctor time was made more efficient."

This was a thrilling result. Howard, Reiffen, Komaroff, and the team were eager to do more, but designing algorithms for diabetes and other medical conditions had revealed a problem: there was an unsettling lack of agreement among very seasoned doctors about how best to take care of patients. This raised an unsettling question: if everyone is doing it differently, can everyone be doing it right? Indeed, what is right? Is there solid clinical science behind the way doctors provide care for a particular medical problem? It was an early premonition of a phenomenon that would become a very important field of health care research beginning about twenty years later: medical practice variation. The team's research demonstrated that doctors treated various conditions the way they were taught to do so even though that training may have taken place two decades earlier, confirming Howard's belief that there was too much art and not enough science in medicine.

"We started out figuring that if you interviewed five diabetes specialists and asked what algorithm should be used for a patient with diabetes—what were the questions you would ask the patients and what was the physical exam involved—that they would all agree," says Komaroff. "But as we talked to doctors it rapidly became clear that, wow, there were lot of different opinions about what was essential or not."

This surprised Komaroff. He had gone into the work believing that specialists in diabetes would share a widely agreed upon method of treatment. "There were a lot of different opinions about what was essential and when we asked people to defend their position, asking what is the evidence to support the value in doing this exam or test, very often there was no evidence at all," he says. "It was just what they thought should be done. There was this remarkable lack of clinical science, more so than any of us would have thought and this was a particular eye-opener for the engineers for whom *everything* was grounded in evidence." It all confirmed Howard's belief that there was too much "art" and not enough science in medical practice.

So Komaroff, Sherman, and their MIT colleagues went back to the drawing board. They conducted a series of studies designed to reveal optimal clinical practice for several of the most common problems in office practice. When a patient presents with a sore throat, for example, how should it be treated? Should everyone get a throat culture? If not everyone, then who? Are the causes of a sore throat always either strep bacteria or a virus as was generally believed, or might other infectious agents be involved? When Komaroff worked his way through the literature he found that in nearly 50 percent of the cases—despite looking for hundreds of bacteria and viruses— there was no apparent cause for a sore throat.

It was not that Howard, Sherman, and Komaroff did not recognize that part of medicine's complexity lies in its hybrid nature as both art *and* science. They very much understood that. But they wanted to push harder on the science side of the equation, always leaving room for individual physician judgment, but in pursuit of as much scientific rigor in the process as possible. This was an important conflict at the time and remains so a half century later. Wide variations in treatment through the years has resulted in uneven delivery and, in some cases, care that is actually dangerous. If there is a best way of inserting and monitoring a central line, for example, shouldn't everyone do it that way all the time? Don't all patients deserve the central line insertion that reduces as much as possible the chances of a deadly infection? This was the direction Howard, Sherman, and their colleagues were headed decades before the kind of standard work recognized today was anything but standard.

As an engineer, Sherman was accustomed to portraying complex problems in the graphic form of an algorithmic tree. This was relatively simple to do with computers, especially the advanced machines Sherman used at Lincoln Laboratory, but those sorts of machines were not widely available and certainly not in a medical center such as Beth Israel. Thus the team worked with paper and pencil.

"I remember vividly," Komaroff recalls, "that when we submitted the first paper about ways in which the use of algorithms to guide the work of non-physician assistants improved the quality of care to the *New England Journal of Medicine*, Franz Ingelfinger, then the editor, said to me, 'This is a clever idea and probably a good one for non-physicians, but this algorithmic approach has absolutely no place in guiding the practice of doctors.' Today, if you open a copy of a textbook for medical students and doctors, such as Harrison's *Textbook of Internal Medicine*, what you see sprinkled throughout the book are the very algorithms that had 'no place' in medicine forty years ago. What was good for non-physicians proved to be good for physicians as well. Sherman deserves recognition for realizing that the concept of systematizing the approach to common problems in medical practice could save money and time—and also improve the quality of care."

As he reflects on it decades later, Komaroff says the work Sherman and his colleagues did was nothing less than groundbreaking. "The most important offshoot of the project with Sherman and MIT Lincoln Lab folks may have been that it played an important role in introducing clinical algorithms into medicine," says Komaroff. "Whereas the algorithms were devised at first for non-physician health professionals, today every textbook for doctors is filled with algorithms." Komaroff notes that some of today's leading voices in healthcare innovation in 2016—Drs. Don Berwick and Atul Gawande, for example—advocate greater standardization. They are seeing "the same lack of systematization in medicine today and saying, 'We need to act more like engineers; we need to be more systematic, for instance, about the procedures we employ in the operating room. What problems are we trying to solve? Sponges have been accidentally left inside a person's body during surgery, requiring new surgery to remove them. Even worse, surgery has been performed on the wrong side: the right knee had the ruptured ligament, but the left knee was operated on. Gawande has demonstrated that checklists that require surgery to be more systematic can reduce these errors. As another example, Berwick has argued we need to be more systematic about how we handle a tube placed into a patient's throat to help him breathe. If it is not handled meticulously, the tube can lead to a lung infection—and people die of that infection. Does being more systematic really matter? The death rate from breathing tube-induced pneumonia used to be approximately 50% but more systematic handling of the tubes dropped the rate to close to zero."

Howard's scientific mind and his openness to collaborating with people like Herb Sherman and Barney Reiffen, suggested his passionate desire to innovate in medicine in different ways. Pushing the innovation envelope was an important part of his job. At the same time, his job required teaching and mentoring young physicians early in their training. An essential aspect to his success in this area came through Howard's personal touch. It is in the nature of academic medicine that doctors and their families pull up roots and move—hundreds of miles, thousands of miles—and get resettled in an entirely new environment. For Howard, making the transition into the BI as seamless and pleasant as possible was a priority. It mattered a great deal to him that his new doctors—and their family members—were comfortable in their new environment. William Silen, MD, the Johnson and Johnson Professor of Surgery, Emeritus, recalls Howard going out of his way to welcome the entire Silen family. Howard had also gone far out of his way to find Silen, talking to people in Colorado in his search for excellence. The welcome included Howard and Doris Hiatt and their children hosting the Silen family at their Brookline home for dinners. "Howard was very welcoming to me and my family," Silen recalled, many decades later. Silen arrived at the BI in 1966 and remained on the Harvard medical faculty until 1995. During Howard's time of leadership at the BI the hospital's reputation grew significantly stronger, recalls Silen. "People regarded it much more highly as time went by," he recalls.

In a time when the vast majority of doctors were white and male, Howard made a point of attracting residents who were neither. Dr. Anne Nicholson, a graduate of University of Pennsylvania Medical School, heard about Howard through a friend who had been chief of medicine at Washington University in St. Louis. The friend told Nicholson that the quality of a medical department depended to a significant extent on the strength of its chief and Howard's reputation had raised the level of the BI programs significantly in just a few years. "When I applied to the BI for an internship it was probably the favored Harvard hospital," says Nicholson. "No, not probably, it was. How-ard had been there five years when I started [1968] and all the major divi-sion chiefs were his picks. They were all young, energetic, and really excited about what they were doing. It was just an amazing environment."

Nicholson and others who worked with Howard at the BI uniformly mention Howard's ability to listen carefully as a key element of his leader-ship style. "I don't know exactly how he picked people," says Nicholson, "but all his division chiefs were extraordinary people. I know he networked a lot and he loved to ask questions and then he really listened. He was a great listener. He was also a wonderful role model for all care-givers: He always spoke to the head nurse and the secretary of the unit before begin-ning rounds, and all of the patients he saw, no matter the diagnosis, felt better after his visit."

Dr. Theodore Steinman, a former professional football player, quarterback for the Detroit Lions, knew what it meant to have your team's full attention. Steinman, who was a resident when Howard was chief of medicine, recalled making rounds with Howard and watching him at the bedside. He would ask questions of the patient and other residents, and "when he listened you could see that the person had his full attention. He was absorbed in what they were saying and I remembered at the time thinking, 'that's the kind of doctor I want to be. I want to have that ability to listen non-judgmentally. He did it in the most natural way."

Howard's desire to listen to other people—patients, family members, staff, physicians—was rooted in his belief that there was great value in what other people had to offer. In an age when some physician leaders believed they were the font of knowledge, Howard believed he had a great deal to learn from others. When he chose young Dr. Wilbert Jordan as a resident at the BI, it was one of the first times the hospital had a black resident. Howard noted in his memoir:

> During my period at Beth Israel Hospital, I grew concerned by the underrepresentation of minority physicians in the Harvard teaching hospitals. There were clearly qualified candidates, but they were being overlooked by the selection committees. As Chairman of Medicine at Beth Israel, when I heard from colleagues about a very promising black fourth year student at Case Western Reserve Medical School named Wilbert Jordan, and heard further that he was applying to our program, I alerted our internship selection committee. We interviewed Wilbert, and over the objections of a small number of the committee members we selected him, and he accepted our offer.
>
> Shortly after his arrival, Wilbert was on duty in the emergency department and was sitting alongside a number of hospital orderlies after a long night. Several were African-American and all, including Wilbert, were in whites. One of our senior physicians came up to him and handed him a tube of blood and said, "Boy, run this up to the lab." "Boy," I subsequently learned, said to this physician, "I am Wilbert Jordan, M.D.," and took the tube to a nearby sink, removed the stopper and poured the blood out. Within a very short time, the senior physician was in my office reporting the story and saying, "I knew we should never have taken him." Next, before I could summon him, Wilbert showed up in my office. "Wilbert," I said, "what have you done to me?" Before answering he volunteered that he was sorry because he knew it meant another stick for the poor patient. "'But,' I recall his saying, 'my sense was that this was an important opportunity to make a statement that would not be forgotten, and that that doctor would never make the same mistake again.'"
>
> It developed that Wilbert played a crucial role in educating both our students and faculty to issues of racism in the three years he was with us. He also played

major role in helping to attract black medical graduates to Harvard teaching hospitals. Later still, he became a leader in addressing HIV/AIDS in Los Angeles. (I was told by a colleague in Los Angeles that he is known as "Dr. AIDS.")

My older son, Jon, who has spent time working on labor problems in Los Angeles, looked up Wilbert on one of his trips. Jon told me the following story. "Wilbert recently was at the airport [in Los Angeles] with time before his flight to Rome and noted that he needed a shoeshine. When he went to the shoeshine stand at the airport he noticed that one of the two seats was occupied, but the person in charge was not there. Wilbert took the other seat and within a short time the other man said to him, 'You know, my flight leaves soon, and I'd be grateful if you could give me a shine.' Wilbert stood up, took a brush and some polish and began working on the man's shoes. Before he had finished the first shoe, the shoeshine man appeared and seemed confused. Wilbert got back in the chair and handed him the brush. The other customer began an abject apology to Wilbert, who told him, "Of course I understand."

Wilbert said to me, 'Tell your Dad this story, and tell him that Wilbert has matured."

In 1971, Jordan noted, Howard was genuinely interested in race relations and he understood the concept that it is a two-way street. There were some white people in positions of power, says Jordan, whose attitude was that they were doing a favor hiring a black person—that "it was a one-way street and only the black person benefitted. Howard was different. He appreciated that there were things I can give you and things you can give me and a lot of the chairs did not get that. When I was a resident he was always very open and receptive and whenever there was an issue I knew I could go and talk with him and I knew he would listen to me."

When Dr. Ted Steinman arrived at Beth Israel for a series of interviews, he was very much hoping to secure a position in the hospital's residency program. As a U.S. Navy doctor who had served in Vietnam, Steinman arrived from Washington wearing his uniform. After meeting with a number of other people at the BI he arrived for his final meeting of the day with Howard, who asked about Steinman's military experience. "Unbeknownst to me at the time, I was in the hotbed of anti-Vietnam movement," Steinman recalls. "Howard's brother Arnold was a major fund raiser for Gene McCarthy's campaign and Howard made it clear that he very much opposed the war. My entire interview consisted of a debate with Howard about Vietnam. When I came back, I was not in favor of the war, but I thought it would be disloyal to speak against the government while wearing the uniform so I was defending the government position and it was a lively debate. Afterward, I flew home to Washington and I told my wife I had the most fascinating interview I ever had but that I will never be accepted. Two days later Howard called me and offered me the position as a second-year resident. I said, 'Dr. Hiatt, I am flattered and I accept. But why, based on our conversation, why am I being offered the position?' And Howard said, 'anyone who can stand up to me and defend their position that well and will not back down I want them here.'"

Howard continually pushed for change at Beth Israel, including for change in sensitive areas. Historically, the hospital had been dominated by outside doctors who held admitting privileges and who treated their own patients while they were in the hospital. There was a clear line of demarcation—medical students could tend to patients on the ward who did not have an outside doctor, but were prohibited from providing care to "private" patients without the explicit approval of the private doctors in charge of the patients. This restricted the ability of the faculty to teach and students to learn. In an effort to improve the scope and quality of education for students, Howard converted the entire medical division of the hospital to a teaching service, thus significantly expanding learning opportunities for residents and medical students and teaching opportunities for faculty. Private physicians outside the hospital were wary of this change, but Howard argued to the hospital's leadership, including the board of trustees, that the change would benefit patients by providing them with continuing care from residents and faculty, thus increasing the chances that their conditions would be expertly monitored. Howard was passionate in his belief that this change was essential if Beth Israel was to rise to the level of quality—in care, education, and teaching—provided by Mass General and Brigham (then Peter Bent Brigham) hospitals. In his memoir, Howard made the case that

> on the ward service, house staff and faculty members were in relationship with patients from time of admission to time of discharge, and representatives were available in the hospital at all times. With the change we proposed, this would now be the case for all patients. Second, separate services had meant that the BI was less attractive to many of the top medical students as a site for training.

While this was a significant cultural change and some private physicians had a reflexively negative initial reaction, after thoughtful discussions the advantages of this approach were obvious. Howard observed in his memoir that with their patients covered by house staff recently out of medical school and supervised by full-time faculty, the private doctors would have the benefit of colleagues with the most up-to-date medical training collaborating on their patient care.... The advantages of coverage by the house staff were doubly convincing with respect to events in the middle of the night: a physician was on hand almost immediately, and there would be no necessity for the private doctors to make their way in to the Hospital in the dead of night—although some, of course, continued to do so.

From a broader perspective, this move was essential for Howard's vision to build a world-class teaching hospital. Recruiting faculty members under the existing, very much restricted structure, would prove difficult. With a commitment to teaching throughout the institution, however, coupled with an effort to advance scientific research, Howard believed he would be able to recruit outstanding faculty.

Change is often difficult in medicine, particularly when it involves making changes to department leadership roles. Tenured medical faculty members sometimes have a tendency to become entrenched through the years and resist anything different from what they are accustomed to. Through happenstance, however, it so happened that a number of chiefs of services at Beth Israel were arriving at retirement age just as Howard was taking over as chief of medicine. Thus, he was in a position to appoint new chiefs and to do so, in most cases, without internal conflict.

During his initial years as chief of medicine, the staff of Beth Israel as well as its board greeted his changes with enthusiasm. He was professional and knowledgeable, but he was also the kind of person to whom others are drawn. There was a charisma to Howard that helped make changes more acceptable to people. Other physicians, students, administrators, board members, and patients saw Howard with his smile and his easy, avuncular manner. He asked about staff member's families and he did so remembering people's names and the names and ages of their kids. He was a rigorous manager but an essential aspect of his management was to connect to people on a human level with warmth, collegiality, and often humor. His self-deprecating brand of off-the-cuff humor became one of his most appealing traits throughout the medical center.

As he worked his way through changes in the early days of his new role, Howard sought the advice of a number of friends and colleagues. In particular, he consulted Dr. Walter Bauer, chairman of the Department of Medicine at Mass General, who had selected excellent young doctors and sent a number of them to NIH for additional training before having them return to Mass General. Given Howard's interest in research, this approach very much appealed to him and he would follow this model at the BI. "I looked for people who were accomplished clinically and very sophisticated scientifically and this was quite unusual," says Howard. A number of well-respected physicians at Beth Israel criticized Howard for this approach, arguing that the goal should be attracting superb clinicians regardless of their research interests or ability. All attention was owed to patients and their ailments, these people argued. But Howard said it was important to take a broader view and that people who were both excellent physicians and accomplished researchers were more likely to identify the best treatments for patients.

As much as Howard loved his work at Beth Israel, he sometimes yearned to get back into the research laboratory. He had experienced the elation of success in the lab years earlier in his work on messenger RNA. There was no feeling quite like the sense of accomplishment that came with breaking new scientific ground. After five years as chief of medicine, with a strong team in place at Beth Israel, he decided the time was right to take a year's sabbatical and immerse himself in the lab. He felt instinctively that it would be impractical to do this in Boston—he knew that if he were on the BI property he would repeatedly be drawn into a wide variety of issues, meetings, decisions to be made. Thus, he took an opportunity to travel to Great Britain to work under a renowned cell biologist at the Imperial Cancer Research Fund Laboratory at Lincoln's Inn Fields in London, one of the world's leading cancer research centers. Howard learned a great deal during his time working with the research scientists. His understanding of cancer deepened considerably.

His work in London also gave him an opportunity to become reacquainted with Dr. Brian Jarman, a general practitioner with a panel of patients mainly in a poor area of London. Many mornings, from nine to eleven, he would make house calls. It was clear the devotion to serving needy patients that Jarman brought to the work. Beyond that, Howard was struck by the power of Jarman's intellect. His preparation for medicine had been quite unusual to say the least. He earned a PhD in geophysics at Cambridge and started out his professional career exploring the Sahara and other deserts for an oil company. He was nearly thirty years old before he started medical school at St. Mary's in London. Howard recalls in his memoir that Brian "spent a summer studying biology on his own and then arrived at St. Mary's to take the battery of entry tests. He had turned in the first test when the supervisor came back into the room to tell him there was no need to go further: he was accepted. After medical school in England he did some training at a London hospital where he impressed the chairman of medicine who called Howard and suggested that Howard accept Jarman into the residency program at Beth Israel. Howard would later tell friends that throughout his career he had many wonderful residents, virtually all of whom, he said, "knew almost as much medicine as I did and one who knew more—Brian Jarman."

What began as a professional relationship between Howard and Jarman evolved into a close friendship between the two men that would stretch over almost six decades. Jarman would go on to become one of the leading primary care physicians in the United Kingdom, head of the Royal College of General Practitioners, and president of the British Medical Association.

The most lasting benefit for Howard from the year in London, in addition to his friendship with Brian, was the opportunity to see the delivery of ambulatory care by the men and women of the British National Health Service. Primary care was Jarman's specialty and he guided Howard through the delivery system with a sense of mission and pride. Howard spent time with Jarman in inner-city London at a clinic serving many working and poor people. He also accompanied Brian on house calls. This effort on the part of Jarman and other NHS physicians to reach out and connect with people in need either through home or clinic visits impressed Howard. There was nothing like this at Beth Israel Hospital.

Thus did Howard become "aware of how much our Department of Medicine and American academic medicine in general were *not* doing, both internally within the hospitals and in surrounding neighborhoods." The National Health Service delivered care to any and all people regardless of their income or social standing and doing so in a setting convenient to the patient left an indelible mark.

Howard returned from London in 1970 with the images of the work he had observed Brian Jarman doing fresh in his mind. He was determined that Beth Israel must do more to provide care to people in need within poor areas of the city of Boston. He also was determined to change the way care was delivered as well as the way the faculty was teaching medical students and residents. This was new ground. Medicine at the time was centered upon treating patients first and foremost and, only then, researching new treatments. Rarely did physicians talk about ways of improving the delivery of care or even what that delivery process should look like. There were standard models—one for ambulatory care and one for in-patient care—and rare was the deviation from these models.

In 1969, while Howard was in London, a radical new experiment in care delivery was launched by a team led by Dr. Robert Ebert, dean of Harvard Medical School. Ebert and his colleagues believed that the best way to deliver care would be through what he called a health maintenance organization (HMO): a group of physicians and other caregivers whose mission would be to keep its members healthy through prevention and early intervention and to provide excellent treatment to those members when they became sick. This HMO model was designed as well to provide care at a lower cost than traditional health insurance plans. Harvard funded this not-for-profit venture, which opened its doors in 1969. From the start, Harvard Community Health Plan attracted talented, idealistic doctors, but its initial efforts to attract subscription-paying members did not fare particularly well. At the start, a grand total of eighty-eight people signed up. Over time, however, the plan flourished.

Ebert also wished to link the new initiative to Harvard teaching hospitals, which Howard thought made perfect sense. Harvard Community Health Plan was unusual for many reasons, not the least of which was its experimental nature. Medicine was then and remains today a conservative profession. Change in healthcare organizations—as we shall see during Howard's years at the Harvard School of Public Health—can be both slow and painful. There is often a predisposition among powerful people in healthcare—including many doctors—to reflexively resist change. Howard recognized, however, that the largely hospital-based model of care was insufficient to meet the needs of many patients in a variety of parts of the community. "What was needed," Howard observed in his memoir, "was a capability within our Department of Medicine to study existing patterns of primary care: How was our society delivering care to people whose medical needs did not require hospitalization?"

> The Beth Israel, like all the other Harvard teaching hospitals, primarily cared for people who had been admitted to the hospital. Its ambulatory care programs served, in general, three categories of patient: patients who did not have a continuing relationship with a doctor; patients who were unhappy with the medical care they were getting and came to the clinic for another opinion; and patients

who were poor, who might also fall into one of the first two categories. For the most part, all these patients came to the Hospital only when they had specific medical problems. When they came, they saw whichever physician happened to be covering at that time.

The question was: Could we study ways in which our society might improve the delivery of medical care for populations like this, using our hospital as the laboratory? To do so, we would want to serve patients who chose to have the hospital as their source of primary care on a continuing basis, not just when they felt unwell.

The result of all this was the creation of the Beth Israel Ambulatory Care program (BIAC), which connected patients with a primary care physician and provided ongoing care to patients via an ambulatory care center at the hospital. Howard was guided and inspired in this work by what he had seen in London. Beyond the ambulatory care center and mindful of Jarman's work in London, Howard established a relationship between Beth Israel Hospital and Dimock Community Health Center in the Roxbury neighborhood of Boston. This was a largely black neighborhood with a good deal of poverty and many health challenges ranging from chronic diseases to gun violence.

Howard was so taken by the work Jarman was doing that he later wrote a column that was published on the op-ed page of the *New York Times* (November 16, 1991) entitled "Meet Dr. Jarman. He makes house calls." The article contrasted the efficiency of the National Health Service with the wasteful nature of delivery in the United States (recounting the story of an elderly man who wanted very much to remain home but who was hospitalized for a series of tests that proved to be not at all helpful medically but nonetheless very expensive). Howard wrote that "Dr. Jarman says that in England ... the continuity of care by general practitioners ... means more prevention and fewer unnecessary procedures, hospitalizations, visits to consultants and costs."

Primary care could do so much more to improve care and control costs but in the United States just 25 percent of physicians are in primary care, while in the UK it is half of all doctors, where their income is on a par with that of heart or brain surgeons. The relationship between primary care doctor and patient is central to the ability of caregivers in the UK to provide ongoing care responsive to patients' overall needs.

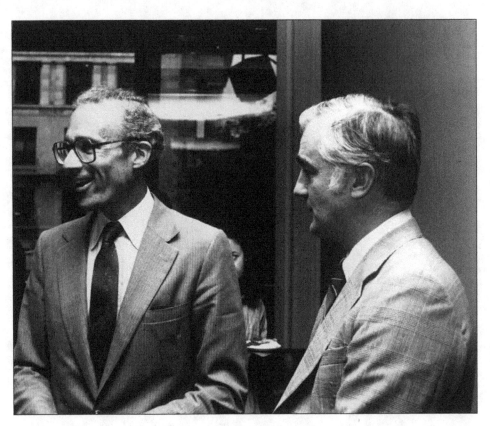

Figure 4.1
Howard Hiatt and Derek Bok.

4 Taking the Leap from Medicine to Public Health

When a smart, charismatic young doctor has as much success as Howard enjoyed building a department at Beth Israel, it does not take long before the suitors from other medical centers arrive at his door. In Howard's case they not only arrived, it seemed at times as though they were lined up outside his door. After he had been chief at Beth Israel for just four years he received a call to determine whether he would be willing to be considered for the position of medical school dean at the University of Rochester. He declined. But an older colleague told him afterward that it was always useful at the very least to go for an initial interview, for if nothing else it could well prove to be a learning experience for both Howard and the institution he was visiting. He took that advice to heart.

Soon thereafter, Howard received an invitation from a physician at Johns Hopkins who was leading a search for a new medical school dean there. This was clearly a very prestigious position but the invitation surprised Howard in large measure because there was a general feeling within the upper reaches of medicine that there was a particular strain of anti-Semitism at Hopkins. But this was one of the most prestigious medical institutions in the world and Howard felt compelled to explore it. He traveled to Baltimore for a series of meetings that went well. Soon thereafter, at a dinner in New York attended by senior faculty members from a variety of medical schools, Howard encountered a doctor from Hopkins. During a cocktail hour prior to dinner "some members drank too much," Howard recalled. "One of these was a Hopkins professor—the person that most of the faculty were said to have considered the likely next dean. He came up to me and told me 'in confidence' that he was certain that I would be unhappy at Hopkins, because too many of the faculty, he said, would be uncomfortable with a Jewish dean. I thanked him for his advice and said that while my mind had not been made up until that evening, this conversation had tipped the scale. I told him that I thought the best way to persuade the kinds of people he was talking about that they were wrong was to take the job and work closely with them."

As discussions continued with Hopkins, there was a recurring theme. Howard was more convinced than ever that major urban medical centers had an obligation to reach out to inner-city communities and provide health-care to poor people and minorities. "But finally, my conversations with several department chairs at Hopkins convinced me that there would be little support for my intention to bring the medical school and the teaching hospital into a closer relationship with the impoverished neighborhood in which they were located. As was the case with so many urban medical schools, there was almost no connection at that time."

A little later, when Howard received a call asking whether he would be willing to be interviewed for the position of dean of Columbia University's College of Physicians and Surgeons (P&S), he agreed. Among the key decision-makers at Columbia were Cyrus Levinthal, a former professor of biology at MIT whom Howard knew, as well as Andrew Cordier, president of Columbia University, and Paul Marks, a friend of Howard's from his time at New York Hospital. From the start, this opportunity looked like something of a slam dunk. Howard was well known to several key decision-makers at Columbia. They wanted him for the job and the Columbia president agreed. And then, very quickly, the whole thing turned upside down.

The weirdness started as soon as Howard was picked up at the airport for his ride into New York City. Howard's friend Paul Marks was nice enough to pick him up, but during the drive Paul "asked me for an assurance that if I took the deanship I would appoint him chair of the Department of Medicine." Howard was taken aback. This was not at all what he considered proper. "I responded that I would surely consider this but could not, of course, make any promises at this stage."

During the course of his first day of meetings Howard felt encouraged. At Beth Israel, he had been working to strengthen the ties between the underserved sections of Boston and his medical center and they had met with some success. A sense of obligation to poor urban communities was central to who Howard was as a physician. This part of the mission in New York seemed particularly significant since there was a large population of poor people in Columbia's back yard. Howard met with the head of Harlem Hospital and with Gordon Chase, commissioner of health for the city of New York, and a former neighbor of Howard's from Worcester. "He and I agreed that there could be a transforming effect on community relations in the upper west side of New York if [Columbia] Presbyterian Hospital, Harlem Hospital, and the community were to seek and find common ground."

This was particularly exciting to Howard. There was something appealing about leading an elite organization such as Columbia into the future, particularly at a time when the cultural and political terrain was shifting so rapidly and significantly in the direction of greater social justice. It all seemed to be lining up nicely. There was only one interview left for Howard to go through, and that was with the head trustee at Presbyterian Hospital, which was closely associated with the School of Physicians and Surgeons. The lead trustee was Gus Long, then president of Texaco. Before speaking with Long, Howard had a conversation with his old friend Alfred Gellhorn at Penn Medical School; he had spent many years on the faculty of Columbia and knew the terrain well. Gellhorn could hear Howard's enthusiasm for the mission of taking care of the community and he cautioned Howard about that. Gellhorn thought Howard was absolutely right in the direction he wanted to go, but "he urged me to be certain that my plans for strengthening the relations in the community were universally agreed upon before accepting the deanship."

Everyone with whom Howard had spoken during the process was on board with the approach—enthusiastic, in fact. Not, it turned out, Gus Long. When Howard told Long of his vision for embracing the local neighborhood, Long responded: "Doctor, our neighborhood is the world. Let me point out to you that the top floor of the ... [hospital] is now occupied by Madame Chiang Kai-shek."

The meeting ended on a chilly note. When Howard called Al Gellhorn, Al suggested Howard withdraw his name from consideration. Howard had the same instinct, but Cyrus Levinthal and Andy Cordier asked Howard to hold off on a decision until he spoke with Gus Long a second time. The next conversation, at Long's home in Florida, seemed to be going reasonably well until Howard turned to potential work in the neighborhood. "I told him again that these issues were crucial to me and said I would take the deanship only with the assurance that he would work with me in the directions that we had earlier discussed," Howard wrote in his memoir. "I had a meeting scheduled with Andy Cordier the next morning, I said, and I needed his advice in advance of my giving Cordier an answer." Long looked at Howard and said, "Doctor, I don't offer advice to anybody."

"On the contrary, Mr. Long," Howard replied. "You have just given me the most forthright advice that I recall ever having received."

Long said to Howard: "My driver is prepared to take you back to the airport when you're ready."

There were other contacts exploring whether Howard might be interested in discussing the possibility of becoming dean at other medical schools. None of these went beyond a few discussions or meetings, until a call from Yale and a series of lengthy conversations with leaders there including the university president, Kingman Brewster. Brewster was an unusual university president in his unabashed liberalism. In the early 1970s, with the Vietnam War raging and the struggle for civil rights resulting in clashes between demonstrators, including members of the Black Panther Party, and police officers, Brewster expressed concern about whether Black Panthers could get a fair trial in New Haven, Connecticut. Brewster was from a well-to-do family in Greater Boston and graduated from the Belmont Hill School before attending Yale, from which he graduated in 1941. He was a naval aviator during World War II, after which he graduated from Harvard Law School (1948). Brewster was keenly tuned in to the zeitgeist of the time and agreed wholeheartedly with Howard's belief that major medical centers had a responsibility to their urban neighbors to provide care to those in need. Brewster so much wanted Howard to come to Yale that Brewster and his wife visited Howard and his wife at their Brookline home to make a formal offer. While he asked Brewster for a week to think it over, Howard had every intention of accepting the position. Howard wrote in his memoir:

> As dean of a medical school, I would be in a position to set up programs that would influence large numbers of physicians early in their medical careers. This would speed the dissemination of the new approaches that had been successful at the B.I. to other hospitals, including outside Boston. I felt strongly that integrating the "new biology" with clinical medicine would produce greater understanding of a range of diseases and, as a result, better care for patients, and I was eager to see that practice spread more widely. I was also convinced that the use of the quantitative analytical sciences to assess the effectiveness of different medical practices ... should be a component of the education of all physicians. This would require adding people with strong backgrounds in the statistical sciences to the traditional medical school faculty. As a dean, I could set up a model of such a move. Finally, I was eager to establish the principle that the clinical concerns of

teaching hospitals should extend beyond the care of hospitalized patients to care of people in the surrounding community, and I wanted to develop more efficient ways of delivering such care. It seemed to me that a medical school deanship would be the natural place to develop and demonstrate leadership in these areas.

While Howard was considering the offer, however, as a courtesy, Brewster called his old Harvard Law School faculty colleague Derek Bok, who had become president of Harvard in 1971 and would remain in that role for twenty years. When he received word from Brewster, Bok set up a meeting with Howard. "Kingman called me to tell me he was hopeful that you would be joining his faculty," Bok said to Howard. "I hope that you will not."

Bok had quite another position in mind for Howard—one of the most challenging jobs anywhere within the sprawling Harvard universe: deanship of the Harvard School of Public Health. Prior to taking office in 1971, Bok had served as dean of Harvard Law School for three years, a role he took on at age thirty-eight. Prior to Bok's taking over, the faculty at the School of Public Health "had just ousted the previous dean, a sign all was not well," Bok recalled during an interview many decades later. During the transition period after Bok was named president but before he had taken office, he received a disturbing report about the school. This came from a "visiting committee," three or four outside experts with ties to Harvard (most were alums) who possessed significant expertise in a particular area. Visiting committees were useful to Harvard administrators in that they provided largely expert and unbiased analysis of how particular parts of the university were functioning. The visiting committee report to Bok concerning the School of Public Health was damning.

"These were well-known scholars, pillars of public health from other schools and their message was quite blunt," Bok recalled. "They said, 'you have a honeymoon period after taking over and our advice is that during that period you should close the school of public health.' They said that it was not up to Harvard standards and 'we don't see a likelihood that it *will be* up to Harvard standards.'"

Before making any decision, Bok spent a couple of days at the school trying to gain an understanding of "what it was about. At that time, the university was very balkanized and as Dean of the school of law I had no idea what the school of public health was up to. I spent two days there and my big impression was the school was involved with some of the most pressing problems in the world including nutrition, the environment, and the economics of healthcare and you can't close a place like that—its agenda is too important."

Bok considered folding it into Harvard Medical School but when he looked at other universities where the public health schools were part of the medical school he found that they were overshadowed by the medical school focus at the time on "science-based acute clinical care of individual patients" and that concentration overwhelmed the public health agenda. "That approach made schools of public health within medical schools second class citizens and that was not the way Harvard should address great problems of the world such as nutrition and the environment and health care policy."

Bok came to the conclusion that the School of Public Health should not be closed, should remain free-standing, and had to be reformed in a major way. "During the fall of my first year I asked the school to set up a committee of senior faculty to do a strategic plan for the school and I met with that committee nearly every week for two to two and a half months and that convinced me that the school in its present guise was incapable of doing a strategic plan. They had no idea how to go about it and what they produced was a pallid reformulation of the status quo."

Bok saw no way to appoint an experienced person from within the school "so I needed to look outside." He had heard about Howard from friends on the Harvard faculty and was aware that Howard had gained a reputation as someone who attracted talented young physicians and researchers to Beth Israel and Bok wanted someone who could do something similar at the School of Public Health. Bok also liked the fact that Howard had broad interests beyond research and clinical medicine and that Howard was interested in and knowledgeable about healthcare policy.

"I knew he had been able to attract younger people who were very bright and were kind of inspired by him to work hard on whatever crusade he was trying to engineer," says Bok. "We had some conversations about him becoming dean and he was excited by the opportunity to build something better." From the very start, says Bok, it was clear that it was "an extremely difficult assignment. We both understood what we were up against."

Howard was taken aback by Bok's offer. He had, as he noted in his memoir, "never set foot in a school of public health." But Bok was convincing and Howard ultimately agreed to take on what would prove to be the most difficult and, at times, the most trying assignment of his career.

"Several of my Harvard Medical School colleagues were puzzled that I would even consider moving to a school of public health," Howard recalled in his private memoir. Many of his friends were surprised while some expressed disbelief. Surely it was a radical departure from the track he was on. And there was some hesitation on his part. Howard was not deeply familiar with the School of Public Health. He hardly knew any faculty members there, and what he knew in general wasn't good.

The opportunity to lead the Harvard School of Public Health into a new era, however, was thrilling. That it was an underperforming member of the elite Harvard community meant that a successful rescue mission would have a great impact on the university and get the attention of healthcare leaders worldwide. More to the point for Howard, however, was his desire to change conditions that affect the health of populations as well as of the individual, and to bring the power of quantitative analytical tools that he believed were underutilized in medicine to public health as well. It could be a chance to convince more and more people in positions of power that there was an obligation on the part of wealthy medical centers to do more to help the residents of urban neighborhoods outside their doors. In many ways, it seemed, the School of Public Health could be an ideal place to accomplish that mission.

Howard was told by Derek Bok that the school was not really a leader in public health and that the faculty in general been there a very long time, had not changed much, and had not kept up with recent developments in science that mattered in public health. Bok wanted Howard to bring the school to the top of the heap, to make it a leader—and that meant bringing change to the school.

Bok believed that Harvard should represent the best—the best of research, the best teaching, the best students. The idea that a Harvard school could be mediocre or only pretty good was something Bok could not tolerate. And the more he looked into the situation at the School of Public Health the more convinced he was that it was average at best and that significant and rapid change was needed.

Howard indicated his forward-thinking nature in an interview with Harvard's student-run newspaper, the *Crimson*, where he said that "over the years there has been a distortion of priorities in the health fields."[1] He cited "the emphasis placed on curative medicine rather than in areas of prevention" and said prevention should become an area of greater concentration among healthcare professionals.

In appointing Howard to the deanship, Bok characterized Howard, according to the *Crimson*, as "a proven administrator and a distinguished clinician and research scholar." Barely a month after Howard was appointed, the *Crimson* noted Bok's seeming propensity to appoint people to leadership positions in a noticeably untraditional manner.[2] The article noted that "President Bok has said repeatedly that he regards appointments as his single most vital responsibility. He puts in a proportionately large amount of time doing background work for the selection of deans and other administrators." The *Crimson* noted that the appointment of a new dean of the Graduate School of Education was unusual in that the new dean "has never had any formal involvement with a school of education. But he has repeatedly proven his administrative ability in government, and he has shown that he can deal successfully with widely different personalities and situations. And that is what Bok looks for in an administrator: experience, tact and proven ability."

The anonymous *Crimson* writer noted that for Bok it seemed that "exact experience in the field is unimportant. Bok's theory is to get the best man available, someone who can overcome a lack of familiarity with the demands of the job and run a division of the University smoothly. This same approach was evident in Bok's choice of Howard Hiatt" to lead the School of Public Health.

Howard noted when he was appointed that because "public health has not been my field," he would "devote the coming months to learning." The *Crimson* article continued:

> Again, the crucial qualification was administrative ability in a related field. Hiatt has successfully guided a large medical staff as physician-in-chief at Boston's Beth Israel Hospital, and Bok obviously figures that the transition to the Public Health School can be accomplished with a minimum of difficulty. The Ed School and the School of Public Health represented two financial problem areas when Bok took over. Apparently the academic precedent of choosing successors from the same field counts for little when Bok gets down to administration.

It is important to place this in the context of previous work Howard had done, particularly leading the department of medicine at Beth Israel. Physicians at the BI saw many patients but there had been little emphasis on research there. Howard changed that and, for the most part, that change was welcomed.

At Beth Israel Howard brought in a team of very young, committed, passionate people who looked up to him as their leader. And when Howard went to HSPH he intended to do something very similar to that. He believed in the pattern of change he had experienced at Beth Israel—bringing in new people with passion and basing the school on hard science, not clinical anecdotes, using an evidence base, a scientific base—and he thought he could change HSPH the same way he had changed Beth Israel Hospital.

Howard's initial discussions with faculty members at the School of Public Health were encouraging. In particular, Jim Whittenberger, chair of the physiology pepartment, expressed concerns about the direction of the school and welcomed the kinds of changes Howard said he hoped to bring about. During a private meeting, Whittenberger "was critical of much that went on [at the school], and his criticisms were in line with many of my own newer impressions. When I described to him some of the things I would hope to do at the School, Jim predicted that the changes I was proposing would be enthusiastically embraced by a majority of faculty. Further, he said that I would have his support for the plans I had outlined."

Howard's feelings at the outset were so positive about Whittenberger that he appointed him associate dean, an effort, Howard noted, to "reassure faculty members who were worried about the "outsider" coming in as dean, and that Jim's presence near the helm would encourage a suspension of doubts while I began making the changes I had in mind."

After taking over in July of 1972, Howard hosted a series of meetings during which chairs of departments from the school would describe the research work within their areas as well as the kinds of courses faculty members were teaching and the content of those courses. At Beth Israel, Howard had come to have the utmost respect for his friends from MIT, Herb Sherman and Barney Reiffen, and Howard asked both men to join him at these informal meetings with HSPH department chairs. It was not that Herb and Barney possessed a particular expertise in public health—they did not. But they had not had expertise in medicine either, yet had played significant roles in improvements at Beth Israel. More than anything, Howard respected their intellectual capacity and trusted their judgments.

"We sat through presentation after presentation," Howard noted in his memoir. "We had come from a department made up largely of young people who were on the cutting edge of work in their fields and excited about future directions, and we found these public health sessions depressing. Had I been exposed to this exercise before accepting the deanship, I would never had done so." During these summer meetings Howard found that much of the research being done "bordered on the trivial, the methodologies were old, and the results were very far from anything that would significantly advance the fields. The biologists among the faculty had no exposure to modern biology, the social scientists other than Alexander Leighton seemed limited in their interests, the work on America's healthcare problems and those of developing countries was pedestrian, there was no research in statistics, the epidemiologists were concerned only with cancer, and the work on diseases of tropical countries seemed to me of limited dimension."

During the first year or so as dean, Howard discovered a professional school lacking in almost every respect. "Why were the people concerned with diseases of the developing world not focusing on the multiple factors resulting from extreme poverty?" he wondered in his memoir. "Why were the laboratory scientists unaware of developments in biological science that might provide new tools for inquiries into (for example) tropical diseases? New techniques were available in computer sciences, offering possibilities for advances in biostatistics and epidemiology, but nobody at the School seemed to be aware of this. The structure of healthcare in the nation was in desperate straits, and yet it was not a topic on the agenda of the Department of Health Services Administration."

In a damning indictment of the school's culture, Howard wrote that "advances in many areas were opening the way to exciting possibilities but, by and large, the faculty of the School of Public Health appeared unaware of new developments in their fields."

Perhaps what set Howard off more than anything else was the siloed nature of the school. It was clear that faculty members were suspicious of people from other disciplines. There was a cultural belief that permeated the school suggesting that anyone not steeped in public health could not make meaningful contributions to the school. This was embodied in the failure of departments throughout the school to engage with other colleagues throughout the university community. "The faculty included people from a range of disciplines, but there was little or no evidence of contact with faculty in the *parent* disciplines in other Schools in the University," Howard wrote. "The professor of health law did not interact with anyone at the Law School; the faculty in the Department of Health Services Administration had no connections with the Department of Economics, the Public Policy program at the Kennedy School or the Business School; the biostatisticians were strangers to Mathematics, and Statistics in the Faculty of Arts and Sciences; the laboratory scientists had not been exposed to modern biology, and so forth."

The state of the school during Howard's initial months was dispiriting. This is not to say that no good work had been or was being done. But the school was tired and insular. The lack of connection with world-class thinkers and researchers in the other professional schools as well as on the faculty of arts and sciences was a failure of vision and demonstrated a lack of energy and even imagination. The interdependent nature of the health of populations whether in wealthy Europe and North America or impoverished parts of Asia and Africa was clear. Health was related to traditional public health areas such as communicable diseases, environment, and sanitation, but it was also clearly related to the law, to businesses and economic factors, and to poverty and education levels. In other words, the work of the School of Public Health was clearly related in many ways to work being done by scholars in virtually every other part of the sprawling Harvard University campus.

Resistance to this notion at the School of Public Health was largely passive prior to Howard's arrival in large measure because no one was pushing the faculty out of their siloes. When Howard arrived, however, resistance to this idea became active and it rested upon a couple of particular pillars that were built up by defenders of the HSPH status quo. In his memoir, Howard noted that in May 1979, he wrote a note for his files in which he stated that upon taking over the deanship of the school, his goals at the outset were first, to bring the social sciences, and particularly the policy sciences, into the School. Second, "I felt that the application of the new concepts and techniques of molecular biology and genetics would have much to offer the public health sciences, and particularly research in the tropical diseases. But beyond all else, it seemed to me that the School was urgently in need of improvement in quality—of its teaching programs, of its research, and of its community activities. It turned out that at the School I was alone in this perception."

In 1972 HSPH had traditional departments such as nutrition, environmental health and sanitation, and tropical medicine focused on parasitic diseases, and the school was training people to run state and local health departments. These departments had not kept up with changes in science. They were weak on basic science. People had been there for a very long time pursuing their own siloed interests and training graduate students in their areas, but they were missing out on huge changes and trends with meaning for public health.

But Harvard was no outlier in this regard. During his first couple of years as dean Howard attended numerous gatherings of leaders and faculty members from other schools of public health from around the country and generally came away struck by the culture of resistance to change and an impulse to cling to the status quo. He was displacing people and bringing in new teachers in each of the main areas of the school. In tropical diseases, he sought a broader approach that would include research and study on HIV/AIDS. In environmental health and toxicology he wanted to measure factory pollution, but he wanted to push beyond that with new approaches to measuring carcinogenicity of harmful chemicals.

Observing Howard's work from across the Charles River (the School of Public Health is located in Boston, not Cambridge), Bok saw that Howard "began very quickly recruiting some very good young people."

Howard had always been a believer that medicine could be more rigorous in measuring quality and effectiveness and he felt that public health also needed a more evidence-based approach. In one of the most interesting personnel moves Howard made, he convinced Fred Mosteller, the all-but-legendary chair of the Department of Statistics in the Faculty of Arts and Sciences, to join the HSPH faculty. Mosteller had the outward appearance of the classic absent-minded professor. He had a casual, easygoing manner, an avuncular nature that drew people to him. Mosteller had gained international renown as a member of the Harvard Faculty of Arts and Sciences for his work in statistics and Howard wanted him to bring his experience and creativity to revamp the public health school's study of biostatistics.

Mosteller had been at Harvard since 1946 and became chair of the new statistics department in 1957. Through the years he and Howard would talk about ways statistics might be applied in medicine, and when Howard took over as dean of HSPH one of his first calls was to seek Fred's guidance in ways to strengthen statistical science within the school. Out of this came many changes, perhaps one of the most important being a regular seminar on statistical methods in public health open to faculty members throughout the university community. This faculty seminar was an early signal of the type of interdisciplinary cross-pollination that Howard wanted to bring to the school. Many prominent professors from different fields—some coming from as far away as Hanover, New Hampshire—attended on a regular basis, although Howard noticed over time "how few seminar participants came from the School of Public Health."

Howard was convinced that healthcare delivery in the United States was performing at a level well below its capability. Yet as Howard looked around the landscape at Harvard and far beyond, he saw little in the way of rigorous study related to how health policy was created and how health delivery systems were managed. This was exciting territory. Howard believed that by marshalling scholars from a variety of disciplines, HSPH could make important contributions defining and measuring the quality and efficiency of care delivery. He wanted HSPH faculty members to collaborate with colleagues from the Harvard Business and Medical schools as well as with scholars on the Faculty of Arts and Sciences in areas of economics, public policy, political science, statistics, and management.

Thus did he create from scratch a Department of Health Policy and Management at the School of Public Health. It was a struggle getting the department off the ground. Howard sought broad faculty support for the new program but it barely squeaked into existence on a vote of the faculty. This was one of the early warnings signaling the insularity of the faculty and the reflexive resistance to change that many of the most senior faculty members would demonstrate throughout Howard's tenure. "It soon became a base for work in a range of areas ranging from healthcare costs to quality of care to the need to make medical services more widely available to impoverished people," Howard wrote.

In addition to training people to work in state and local health departments, the idea was to bring modern management practices to the delivery of health services. Howard wanted to improve all of the parts of the healthcare system by adapting new management approaches as well as quantitative science to measure clinical and cost effectiveness. None of these new health policy and management practices was being incorporated. The new curriculum included courses in biostatistics, health economics, cost accounting, and clinical operations management.

The Department of Health Policy and Management was designed to examine and challenge existing methods of care delivery in the U.S. "There were few things I felt more strongly about than the urgent need for changes in the American health care system," Howard wrote in his memoir. "So much was being lost in terms of both money and quality because of unexamined medical practices that were being continued almost by rote."

To change the system of care delivery it was necessary to provide leaders in healthcare with the managerial tools they needed to make these changes. "I knew that I myself had assumed the role of chair of a department of medicine—which is, in addition to its medical component, a managerial role—without an adequate background in policy or in management," Howard wrote. "In fact, I had no background at all in those areas, and I knew the same was true for virtually all of my colleagues who chaired clinical departments and for most deans of medical schools as well. You learned on the job or you didn't; it came quickly or it didn't."

> To establish a home for these executive programs, I put forward at a faculty meeting my proposal for a new department at the School to be called Health Policy and Management. The faculty was deeply divided on the proposal. ... I believed that in many cases it sprang from honestly held opinions that reflected true disagreement about the boundaries and concerns of public health. But I also believed that those opinions were rooted in the characteristic unwillingness to entertain new ideas that I was regularly encountering at the School. ... Though by a narrow margin, a department that would become a model and then a staple for schools of public health, even including the name, was voted in.
>
> An area that seemed particularly suited to collaborative attention was environmental health. With initial funding from the Environmental Protection Agency and the Mellon Foundation, I set up the Interdisciplinary Programs in Health (IPH). Like the Center for the Analysis of Health Practices (CAHP) and the Executive Programs in Health Policy and Management, IPH was based in the Dean's Office.

Howard frequently spent time talking with friends and colleagues in other parts of the university, including John McArthur, dean of the Harvard Business School. In carrying out Derek Bok's charge to put HSPH on the map, Howard wanted to understand how other Harvard professional schools had sustained their influence. McArthur told Howard that an important component of the Business School's clout was the impact of its many executive education programs. In addition to training graduate business students, the school also hosted a variety of programs for executives from companies throughout the world in all manner of industries. This meant that the B school faculty was in constant and close touch with leading executives and thus was learning what was going on inside companies. It also meant that the Harvard faculty could influence the very men and women who held power in some of the world's great companies.

The idea that executives from major companies would make their way back to Cambridge for refresher courses was telling. These were managers with a strong business school foundation and years if not decades of managerial experience. This was in sharp contrast to the lack of managerial training that most physicians have when they take over large departments or medical centers. "I knew firsthand how little in the way of managerial and administrative background I had when I took over as chairman of the department of medicine and many of my colleagues in similar jobs around Boston and around the country had a similar lack of preparation and experience." Asking physician leaders to take off a few months or even weeks would not work, in Howard's view, but a program offered a couple of afternoons a week might draw in health leaders seeking administrative and leadership capability. Thus, he established an executive program within the new division of Health Policy and Management with the goal of connecting with healthcare professionals in the same way the business school connected with business executives. Howard secured several million dollars in funding for these programs from the U.S. Department of Health, Education and Welfare under the Nixon administration. Getting this government funding for the executive education programs was quite a coup—and quite resented by other schools of public health. He offered innovative afternoon courses for leaders in a variety of subjects including statistics, management practices, and administration. These courses, which would prove to be among the most popular at the School of Public Health, also served to build closer ties between a number of other graduate schools and HSPH.

Intellectual cross-pollination was among Howard's most powerful beliefs. He was convinced that when powerful minds were brought together—experts in a wide variety of not obviously connected fields—that connections and relationships would become visible and that great things were possible.

This approach, however, collided head-on with the widespread belief throughout the faculty that training in public health was a prerequisite to being able to provide valuable insights at the school. "The concept of 'knowing public health' was the basis not only for acceptance but also for exclusion," Howard wrote in his memoir. Among the most egregious examples of this narrow thinking was the appointment of John Cairns, a molecular biologist whom Howard had known from his research stint in London. Cairns was, by any measure, a giant in the field, a world-renowned molecular biologist with a deep knowledge of cancer. He had been offered tenured appointments at Harvard College and Harvard Medical School and turned down both. But he was excited by Howard's vision for HSPH and, at Howard's urging, agreed to join the faculty there. "Cairns was looking to combine molecular biology with public health, broadly defined, taking it in new directions," Howard wrote. Where, exactly, would this lead? It was unclear, but that was sometimes the nature of research. The idea of letting Cairns loose within the school and letting his powerful mind seek to make connections was truly exciting to Howard. The reaction to what would be widely seen as a coup for the school from much of the senior faculty was, "What does he know about public health?" They would have turned him away.

John Cairns came to the school and made a profound impression on many of the young faculty and students. His interests were wide, his knowledge in areas beyond his own specialties was extraordinary, and his eagerness to help young people was apparent. One of the young scientists then at the school said "John has the uncanny ability to understand deeply everyone else's research, whether it's in his field or not. I didn't believe this when I first heard of it from others, but I became a believer when he instantly recognized some arcane feature in my acid rain data that I hadn't even thought to pursue."

For the school, John functioned as a scientific beacon. He was willing to give advice and counsel. Molecular biologists in other Harvard schools found him a kindred spirit, and because of his connections with them and other scientists, the school's agenda became better known in other parts of the university. Was this the traditional public health model? Certainly not, but if Derek Bok had wanted the traditional public health model he would not have asked Howard to take over as dean of the school. And if the traditional public health model had been the goal, Howard would never have accepted the position. Greatness for HSPH was achievable not through the traditional health model but by exploring new connections; by taking risks; by having the courage to do things differently; by bringing exceptionally talented people together and seeing what emerged.

The reaction to the Cairns appointment, however, was depressingly predictable: "What," leading faculty members asked, "does he know about public health?"

One of his earliest initiatives at HSPH was establishing what he called the Center for the Analysis of Health Practices, which provided a formal structure within which cross-pollination could occur. CAHP "evolved from conversations initiated by Herb Sherman and others about applying analytical tools that cut across the disciplines of medicine, epidemiology, biostatistics, economics, the social sciences and engineering to challenges in health and medicine. The mix of individuals who would be required to team up to address these problems did not comfortably fit into any of the traditional departments of the School." Howard's work reshaped most of the major departments at the school and established interdepartmental connections and collaboration as the preferred way of doing business.

By the time he took over as dean, Howard had been at Harvard in one way or another for thirty years! And through those years he had made it his business to get to know many different faculty members from a wide variety of departments throughout the university. He had many good friends at the medical school, of course, but he also had close friends at the law and business schools as well as on the faculty of arts and sciences. This familiarity proved an enormous benefit in his desire to inject new energy and ideas into the School of Public Health. "To reach beyond the traditional public health community, I assembled a list of advisors and talent scouts," a group of creative and engaged scholars from outside the school. These included, among others, the economists Howard Raiffa and Thomas Schelling at the Kennedy School; Martin Feldstein in the Department of Economics; Jim Vorenberg, Frank Sander, and Charles Fried at the Law School; Larry Fouraker and John McArthur at the Business School; Matt Meselson, Konrad Bloch, Wally Gilbert, Frank Westheimer, and several others in science departments at FAS; and a large number of former colleagues at the Medical School. Many of these talented people played a role at HSPH either through informal discussions with Howard or through regular contributions at CAHP sessions.

Even as he was organizing CAHP, there were signs of trouble ahead. Many veteran faculty members at the school felt that from the start Howard was leading the school in a new and inappropriate direction. And when Howard brought in people with diverse backgrounds who were not an obvious and comfortable fit within a traditional public health structure, existing department chairs refused to find room in their departments. "A number of the people I had recruited had been rejected for membership by department chairs and needed an academic home. For this reason, CAHP was set up as a program in the Dean's Office." Howard was able to recruit another distinguished scientist, Don Hornig, who had been president of Brown University and science advisor to President Lyndon B. Johnson.

Tension between Howard and the faculty grew with each new initiative he suggested. He wanted change and more rigorous science and stronger connections to other areas of the university. The faculty wanted people with little or no training in public health to stop interfering in their research and teaching. While School of Public Health faculty viewed experts in other fields as alien to their field of expertise, Howard was convinced integration of ideas was the sine qua non of the school's potential excellence.

There were two ways to look at a number of early initiatives by Howard, CAHP included. Viewed from one perspective the new department within the Dean's office brought together great minds pushing for innovative solutions to a wide variety of challenges in public health. Viewed from another perspective, the creation of the department was viewed with suspicion by established HSPH faculty who felt a growing sense of mistrust in their new dean. This compounded resentment and distrust that may have had its origins in the way Howard had been selected: Derek Bok had chosen Howard himself without soliciting faculty input through a search committee. The fact that Bok conducted all of his dean appointments this way would probably not have made faculty resent this any less.

An early and defining example of the growing mistrust came as a result of a phone call from Howard Raiffa, an expert in decision science and a professor of managerial economics at both the Business and Kennedy Schools. "Howard called me one day to say that he thought decision science had much to offer medicine and public health," recalls Howard. "He told me he had a student named Milton Weinstein, a very gifted young man about to get his Ph.D. at the Kennedy School, who was interested in applying the techniques to medical and health issues. I interviewed Milt and was greatly impressed. I described him—with Raiffa's evaluation—to the then heads of the [HSPH] departments of Biostatistics, Epidemiology, and Health Services Administration, saying that I would find the resources if they would like to offer him an appointment in one of their departments."

But none of these department heads wanted Weinstein. None saw any value in his ability and credentials within public health in general or their departments in particular. It was this kind of siloed, narrow thinking that was immensely frustrating to Howard, for it was the polar opposite of the way he thought. Howard brought Weinstein into CAHP and he went on to play a defining role in the school as a pioneer in clinical decision-making and clinical effectiveness.

Howard obtained foundation grants to fund CAHP within the office of the dean. Milt Weinstein was one of many appointees within the department including Herb Sherman and Barney Reiffen as well as a number of young Harvard Medical School–trained physicians who had also studied public policy at the Kennedy School. Two of these young doctors—Harvey Fineberg and Don Berwick—would go on to become some of the most important leaders in healthcare and public health in the late twentieth and early twenty-first centuries.

Howard had been quite successful in leading change at Beth Israel Hospital. He approached the job at HSPH in a similar way, yet the two institutions were very different. "The Beth Israel was a small place with a small number of tenured faculty and a lot of private and federal money to grow," says Dr. Tony Komaroff. "In contrast, while there were many outstanding faculty at HSPH, there was also some 'tenured deadwood'— faculty who had made important contributions in the past, but no longer and who remained somewhat aloof from the work of the school. "There was a problem with lack of rigor among some tenured older faculty members." The problem was compounded by the school's practice of awarding "administrative tenure," a process quite different from the rest of Harvard University with a less-than-rigorous search and the necessity for these tenured faculty to raise their own salary.

Howard expressed deep concern about the maldistribution of resources within healthcare in the United States, but a number of faculty members at the School of Public Health thought that investing time in such public policy areas was inappropriate for a public health school. Yet Howard believed that the school's statisticians, sociologists, and other experts could delve more deeply into the study of benefit versus cost and benefit versus risk. In studying these areas additional help and insight could come from faculty at the business, law, and other schools in the university.

In each of the major areas within the School of Public Health Howard tried to bring new, evidence-based approaches to studying and implementing public health practices. Faculty saw these changes as threats to their domain. Many of these faculty members had been there a very long time and wanted to continue to do as they pleased because they were tenured. Howard felt he had orders from Bok to make quick changes at the school and he sought to make some very big changes very quickly. He ran into a lot of entrenched faculty members who told him "not so fast. You're not even a public health practitioner. You're a medical doctor." Many faculty rebelled against him outright.

Howard wasn't used to having people resist him. He was used to having people praise him. At Beth Israel people appreciated what he did. At the BI he made significant personnel changes. He pruned to grow. Sometimes you have to cut bushes way, way back to get them to grow and flourish and that's what he had done at the BI and sought to do at the School of Public Health.

Howard loved Harvard. He had loved it as a seventeen-year-old undergraduate, as a medical student, and as head of the Department of Medicine at a Harvard teaching hospital, and he had always held an unshakable belief that Harvard should always represent the best; the best scholars, researchers, teachers, students. Harvard had opened doors for Howard at some of the elite centers of scientific and medical research in the world including NIH and Pasteur. Harvard had helped raise Howard's reputation throughout the country and drawn the interest of many different medical schools with an interest in having someone of his stature as dean. He had little patience for mediocrity and he was taken aback at the lack of quality within HSPH. He was empowered by no less than the president of the university to step in and forge a new direction; to elevate HSPH to the upper ranks of public health schools in the world. That was the Harvard way, he believed, and aspiring to anything less than the best would be to capitulate to the avatars of mediocrity who seemed to populate the school. A lot of the faculty had been there a long time and had committed a lot of time and effort to the school and felt their chairs, their departments, and their disciplines were theirs to do with as they thought best. And now the new dean comes in and says we need to make changes and get this place up to date and up to snuff.

From across the river, Bok was aware of the challenges Howard faced. "Inevitably some eggs had to be broken not only to bring in young people," says Bok, "but also some of the existing people came up for tenure and Howard with my enthusiastic encouragement applied high standards from the rest of the university which meant a number of these people got turned down. The impression that got around in the school of public health was that Howard really didn't think the standards were what they ought to be and some pretty drastic measures were necessary over time to bring it up to speed. That did not endear him to people at the school who felt they were doing just fine thank you."

In his memoir, Howard identified two notable elements of the defense of the status quo, including "exclusion of those with different training." The sense among the faculty was that unless one was trained in public health, one had no business being in any position of authority at the school. This spoke to the narrow definition of the discipline. Some physicians at Beth Israel had objected when Howard had brought in Herb Sherman and the team from Lincoln Laboratory at MIT. "What do engineers know about medicine?" they asked, albeit in generally quiet tones. The answer was: "Let's explore and find out." Doctors at the BI were a curious lot and had been happy to go along with that experiment, which yielded important results.

But that kind of thinking was largely absent from the School of Public Health. It was as though being an MD, not a PhD in public health, meant that as Howard walked from the dugout to home plate for his turn at bat, he already had two strikes on him—different standards and different training.

Howard also faced unwillingness on the part of existing faculty to "accept new approaches"; to try new ideas. This was the antithesis of Howard's approach to solving problems. It was the antithesis of what he had done at Beth Israel; the antithesis of the culture and attitude he had sought to instill at the BI. "I ultimately concluded," Howard wrote in his memoir, "that when public health people posed the question, "What does he know about public health?" what they were asking was whether the person in question had been in a school of public health. It was a self-referential loop, a way of keeping people (and ideas) out."

There was a particular incident that brought this attitude to the fore while causing a rift between Howard and many members of the school's faculty. A professor in the toxicology division of the physiology department was up for tenure. As with any initiative for tenure throughout the university, the process was initiated by the chairman of the department in which the candidate for tenure worked. At that point, however, the process at the School of Public Health diverged from the tenure pathway followed throughout most of the rest of the university.

Rather than to an *ad hoc* committee made up of experts in the candidate's field and related areas from both within and without the University, as was the case in other schools, nominations for tenured positions at the School of Public Health proceeded to the School's Administrative Board, which was comprised of the chairs of School departments. Thus, not only was a candidate's work judged by people who, in many cases, had little or no familiarity with his or her area of scholarship, but each chairperson knew that next time his or her own candidate would be subjected to a similar process. The opportunities for decisions based on other than the academic merits of the candidate were evident. And such was the state of tenure at the School of Public Health that, I was told, two professors in the Department of Tropical Public Health had been granted tenure with *no* committee review at all, because the dean at the time had convinced the Harvard president that there were no scholars capable of evaluating their work. I would become very familiar with this mantra: Only public health experts know public health.

Howard wanted a more rigorous vetting process and Derek Bok agreed with him. A committee of experts was appointed, including a Nobel laureate in chemistry. The professor up for tenure in toxicology was well liked among colleagues throughout the School of Public Health, where the notion that outsiders were intruding in their area of expertise seemed to grow stronger each day, and the issue of this tenure decision took on great significance. When the review committee deemed his research insufficiently rigorous, he was turned down, and a wave of faculty anger crashed down upon Howard. The head of the department in which the division of toxicology was located asked Howard, "What do we do now? Are you going to close Toxicology? This man is head of the national academy of toxicology. You won't find a better toxicologist." Ultimately Howard found a superb person to head this department in Armen Tashjian, a professor at Harvard Medical School, who transformed the field of toxicology from dosing rats and observing the results to chemical and biological investigation of the substances in question.

Howard was very smart and precocious. He skipped grades in school, started medical school before finishing college. He was used to solving problems using his head, an approach that is very good for solving scientific problems but not always so good for solving problems dealing with people. People don't always behave by rational scientific principles. Howard did very well at Beth Israel Hospital, but at the Harvard School of Public Health he ran into the type of problems that just being smart doesn't help you solve or understand. He didn't understand why there was such strong resistance and opposition to what he wanted to do. He felt he was going in on his boss's orders, and knowing that, people would comply because he had the backing of the president. But it was an entrenched faculty with tenure and they weren't to be bossed around by anyone. Howard did not understand how fiercely the faculty members believed they had earned the right to be totally independent and tenured and in their chairs forever. Howard had never encountered that kind of resistance.

Howard operated by doing nice things for people and it worked wonders. People were very appreciative of what he did for them. But he did not understand what a threat he represented to other people, and when feeling threatened, people react very differently. He was not prepared to understand that or deal with it in a very effective way.

A consensus emerged among faculty members opposed to much of what Howard was doing. They believed that the appointment of someone without extensive public health training and experience was a terrible mistake. They believed they understood the field by nature of their extensive training, research, and practical experience. They believed absolutely that they had, collectively and individually, been engaged in doing the right research and teaching the right courses.

They felt Howard condescended to them, that he did not take the time to listen to and understand them. Many expected him to come to the school and invest time in learning what they were doing and yet, from their perspective, he did the opposite: He plowed ahead with change they considered ill-advised, abrupt, and far too rapid.

As dean, Howard had a "disdain for mediocrity," in the words of Don Berwick. Howard, Berwick noted, was something of an intellectual elitist who was unable to "tolerate a certain kind of mediocrity of intellectual contribution."

Howard never regretted accepting the appointment as dean. He did, however, regret not making an arrangement with Derek Bok to make sure Howard would have the funding needed to hire a world class faculty. "When Derek recruited me to make major change, I should have asked him to assure me specifically of his help in raising the money that would be required."

Had I been a savvier academic administrator, more aware of the fiscal realities of universities (as opposed to hospitals) and of the costs of the programs I considered essential, I might have made that a condition of my acceptance. Because I did not do so, I was largely on my own in finding money for what was needed to change the institution. And since alumni of schools of public health are not, in general, made rich by the careers that await them, the search for serious resources had to be undertaken among people who knew little or nothing about such schools. This proved to be time-consuming, and worse, it was often unsuccessful. Lack of resources made it difficult or impossible to recruit senior faculty to head programs that were taking new directions, which might have made acceptance of these programs more likely. As it was, the increased focus on obtaining resources for new efforts caused resentment at the School. Many of the faculty questioned why the new dean was spending so much time seeking support for initiatives that seemed to them to have little relevance to public health rather than helping them find funding for their work (work for which, in many cases, I could not in good conscience have asked for support).

Howard was actually challenging the faculty on two fronts, substance and procedure. He had made it clear that the tenure situation (procedure) had perpetuated the general mediocrity and prolonged the failure to keep up with scientific advances in the disciplines pertinent to public health. As a result, the substance of what he was trying to do (bring public health into communication with new science and technology) threatened their deeply held concepts of what public health was. He was coming at them on both fronts, as they saw it. That Howard had also made known among HSPH faculty that he intended to stay for only five years was, in retrospect, a mistake, for it effectively made him a lame duck in the eyes of the faculty from the beginning.

Life at the School was very different from what I had known before at Beth Israel. When I was at the BI, if I were unaccompanied on my morning walk from Brookline I would turn over in my mind what lay ahead that day, and I would be filled with anticipation and enthusiasm as I walked. I imagine there might have been a little bounce to my step as I made my way to Morning Report. When I walked to the School of Public Health in the mornings it was a very different experience. Trudging, not bouncing, would describe my step, and after the first couple of years, through my head ran over and over the question, "Why did I take this job? What have I gotten myself into?"

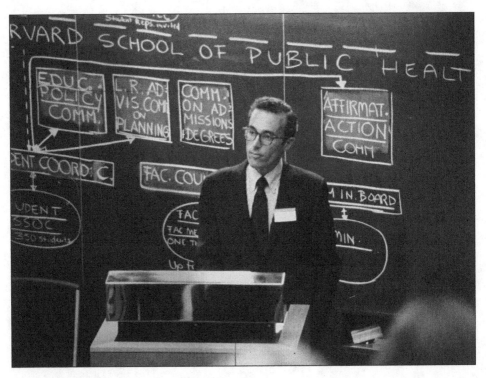

Figure 5.1
Howard discussing plans for reorganization at the Harvard School of Public Health.

5   A Brewing Storm

The contrast between Howard's prior experiences and the situation he faced at the School of Public Health was stark. Throughout his career—ever since entering Harvard College as a seventeen-year-old—things had gone well for Howard. Extremely well, in fact. He had been capable of starting medical school after only a year and a half of undergraduate study and after his training he had conducted research at NIH and the Pasteur Institute alongside scientists who were giants in their field. He had been welcomed and valued at every step along his career path, never more so than when he was made chief of medicine at the BI. His professional trajectory was quite remarkable. On the verge of becoming dean of Yale Medical School, he had been wooed by no less a personage than the president of Harvard University. *Don't leave, Howard, you are too valuable here at Harvard. I need you for one of the most challenging and important assignments within the university.*

Howard responded to the call of duty from Bok with energy and enthusiasm—and, perhaps most important, with an expectation that things would go as well at the School of Public Health as they had always gone for him. Howard had, in a way, a golden touch. It was the combination of his personal charm and approachable manner coupled with an extraordinary mind, clear vision, and a fierce tenacity. Howard Hiatt had gotten along with virtually everyone he had ever worked with. He was kind and, much as anything else, he possessed a big heart. He cared about people. He sought to help others whenever possible. All of this should have made for a relatively smooth ride at HSPH. But the reality is that Howard had to fight for every change he made. He faced opposition to virtually every decision he made. And the fundamental reality was that the key players on the SPH faculty did not want to change—at least not much. Revisions around the edges, at the margins, that they would tolerate, but the faculty made it clear they would oppose Howard on any and every major change. In Howard's view he was up against "resistance that was grounded in self-interest. Partly because of the anomalous tenure process ('you scratch my back ...') and the associated need to raise their own salaries, the chairs of departments at SPH were like medieval barons, each with his (or her) own fief. The best example would be the head of nutrition, the biggest money-raiser at the School, who had gotten millions from cereal companies and, most egregiously, from the sugar people. He had the largest building at SPH, for which he had raised all the money. Only this past year—40 years later—there was a news story about how nutrition research had been deliberately misreported, maybe even faked, to identify fat rather than sugar as the main dietary threat—this reporting came from HSPH professors and influenced the 'food pyramid' recommendations of the US government for years." This predated Howard, but in his eyes it was "an example, though extreme, of the kind of autonomy the 'barons' expected. Apparently there was no possibility for reining in this kind of misinformation coming out with the imprimatur of a Harvard School. The barons were untouchable—and wanted to remain so."

Howard for his part carried with him an assignment from the university president. This was his cudgel. The mission from Bok gave him the certainty he needed to forge ahead with widespread change. But it was ugly. "Every proposed change was confrontational from start to finish," Howard later wrote. "Most of the senior faculty who were at the school when I arrived were adamant in their opposition to the changes I wanted to make.... The result was a climate of frustration and bad feeling."

Five years into his tenure at the school Howard was deeply frustrated. While he had been able to accomplish some important moves—such as instituting a rigorous search process for tenure decisions, building a first-rate biostatistics department, starting a new department of health policy and management that brought to the school quantitative and qualitative analytic skills that could be focused on improving healthcare in the United States, and attracting world-class scientists to the school—every step had been a slog through the mud against resistance. Then, when Bok appointed a new dean of the Harvard Medical School in 1977 without conferring with Howard in advance, Howard was furious. Bok, he said, had "promised repeatedly that he would consult with me before the medical school deanship changed hands. I believed this was crucial, because the good will and cooperation of the dean of the medical school were so important to the School of Public Health."

In fact, Howard thought Bok's choice of Dan Tosteson was excellent, but Bok had no way of knowing Howard's feelings. Howard and Dan had been medical school classmates and were good friends. In addition, Howard had already decided that he would take his exit after five years as dean, as he had told Bok he would when he took the job. He planned to resign the following year. But this oversight by Bok strengthened his resolve. He thought that it could well be interpreted by HSPH faculty as a loss of confidence and support on Bok's part. With that support in question, further changes at the school would be all but impossible. During a meeting in Bok's office, Howard expressed his disappointment in not being consulted on the new dean of the medical school and told Bok he intended to resign as dean of the School of Public Health. Bok "apologized profusely and pleaded with me to change my mind," Howard wrote in his memoir.

Bok does not recall this meeting, although he says it might well have taken place just as Howard describes. "I don't remember that," says Bok, "although it would not have surprised me." The situation at the School of Public Health was not going to be solved easily. "I knew there would be moments where one might despair about getting this millstone from one's neck, but I would have urged him to stay on, because progress was being made."

Howard's recollection is that during the course of a Friday afternoon meeting, Bok called for a timeout and asked Howard to meet him back in his office the following morning, a Saturday. Howard returned to Harvard Square the next day and met with Bok, who said that it was extremely important that Howard remain as dean and continue working toward the goals "you and I have shared." The intensity of Bok's appeal was indicated by the fact that for part of the session the president of Harvard sat on the arm of Howard's chair, appealing to Howard's sense of mission. Bok mentioned several brilliant young or new faculty members being mentored at the school by Howard and asked what would happen to them if Howard left? Howard was struck by this. He felt a commitment to the people he had recruited—Harvey Fineberg, Don Berwick, Milt Weinstein, Herb Sherman, Barney Reiffen, and many others. He had built something special, a team of people who were doing important research and teaching. Bok said he believed Howard had a moral obligation to stick by his team, and Howard could not disagree. It was, Howard wrote, "the one argument that I could not dismiss." He told Bok he would stay on. But privately, he was not happy about it. And things only deteriorated from that point forward.

In June 1978, six years into Howard's tenure as dean, the faculty of the School of Public Health realized that five years had gone by and there was no sign of their dean leaving, as he had said he would consider doing when he arrived. While Howard and Doris were on a post-commencement vacation on the rivers of France with their good friends Jim Vorenberg, the dean of the Harvard Law School, and his wife, Betty, there was an open revolt among a number of senior faculty members. Seventeen of the thirty-four tenured faculty at the School signed a petition to Bok seeking Howard's removal. Bok received the petition on June 19. Three other senior or recently retired professors wrote letters to Bok also seeking Howard's removal. Howard received this news while calling in to his office from a phone booth in France. Howard was extremely upset by the letter. He wanted to return immediately, but his friend Jim Vorenberg persuaded him to continue on the trip and to try and relax as much as possible before going back to face the storm. "I am your lawyer," Vorenberg said. "You will stay here and finish your vacation."

When he returned from vacation, Howard was told that Bok would speak with him after he had spoken with the each of the letter writers who wished to see him and would then make a decision about the matter. Howard wrote in his memoir that

> To say that these next weeks were the most difficult time of my academic life would be to understate it. The period of limbo over the summer while Derek talked and pondered seemed interminable. The irony of it did not escape me. One year before I had gone to Bok to tell him that I was resigning, and he had pleaded with me not to go. Now, I was determined not to resign while he decided whether to ask me to leave.

The bitterness toward Howard spilled over into the press when several faculty members at the School of Public Health went to a reporter at the *Boston Globe* and informed her of the petition seeking Howard's removal as dean. On August 14, 1978, *Globe* medical reporter Loretta McLaughlin wrote a piece that was largely uncritical in reflecting the views of the signers of the letter to the president:

> A faculty revolt at Harvard, unprecedented in scale and in the professional stature of the professors involved, has erupted at the university's prestigious School of Public Health....
>
> The petitioners hold Hiatt responsible for the school's accreditation now being "in jeopardy," the school's increasingly "precarious financial position," and the

alienation of previously generous private donors and foundations at a time when a \$40 million endowment drive is to be launched.

The article noted that signers of the petition "would not have been moved to such action were it not for 'intolerable provocation,'" which they indicated included Howard's "administrative ineptitude," and his "constant deprecation of the quality of our students and of the faculty." The reporter called Howard to respond to her questions; she quoted him in the article as indicating that there was resistance from the "old guard" to change. "Change is difficult," he told her. "I believe we're doing what society demands, and that is difficult for many of them on the faculty. I'm sorry about that."

Deteriorating relationships within SPH were bad enough. The personal enmity toward Howard among some faculty members was deeply unpleasant. But to have the entire matter now splashed across the front page of the newspaper made it all uglier still. "For the quarrel to have progressed to a showdown is virtually unheard of within Harvard academic circles where such matters traditionally are settled behind closed doors," the article stated.

Howard responded to the moves against him by pulling together a group of trusted friends and advisors and working out a strategy to blunt faculty criticisms and keep his job. One of the most striking aspects of the faculty revolt was that it represented a point of view about Howard that was the polar opposite of how many other faculty and administrators at the university viewed him. Throughout his time at the university—as an undergraduate, in medical school, during training, and at Beth Israel Hospital, Howard was well respected and well liked. Thus, the faculty revolt was something Howard had never before experienced in his life. In fact, it may have been the most forbidding obstacle that Howard had ever encountered. "It was the first wall he had ever hit," recalls his brother Arnold. "Howard was a golden boy when he took over at the School of Public Health. I'm not sure he ever experienced great disappointment in his life before that. I think he had more confidence than he should have. I was concerned with the pace at which he was changing the school."

During this difficult summer Howard awaited word of his fate from Bok. Never before had Howard experienced anything like the unpleasant mix of anxiety, frustration, and anger that he experienced during those sultry months. Add fear and embarrassment to the mix and it became toxic—fear for his reputation and embarrassment at being publicly humiliated within the institution he so revered and to which he had given so much.

During this time Howard received an invitation to lunch from Thomas D. Cabot, a man who was as much Mr. Harvard as anyone since John Harvard himself. Cabot was from the elite Boston family—the expression was that "the Lowells speak only to Cabots, and the Cabots speak only to God." Thomas D. Cabot had been director of the Harvard alumni association, served on the board of overseers of the university, and donated the funds for the Harvard Cabot Science Complex; other facilities at the university bore the Cabot name as well. Just a few years prior to sitting down to lunch with Howard, Cabot had been awarded an honorary degree as well as the Harvard Medal.

After a brief interval of small talk, Cabot got to the point: "I want to tell you something that might help you make a decision," he said, according to Howard's recollection (Cabot died in 1995). Cabot explained that while he was serving on the Harvard board of overseers he also held the position of chairman of United Fruit at a time in the 1960s and early 1970s when a number of critical articles were written about the company's treatment of workers throughout its vast holdings in Central and South America. The charges involved exploitation of workers and land by United Fruit and corruption through bribery of government and regulatory officials. United Fruit at the time became a symbol of the sort of colonialism that the political left in the United States and Europe found particularly objectionable. Cabot told Howard that as chairman of United Fruit he felt at a certain point that the criticism of the corporation was reflecting badly on Harvard, given his position on the board of overseers. With so much negative publicity about the company, usually with Cabot's name included, he told Howard that he felt he had a decision to make. Harvard's name came into play in articles where it was noted the position Cabot held at Harvard and that concerned him.

"I thought about how to handle this because I did not want the Harvard name to suffer," he told Howard. "I decided the best way to handle the situation to make sure the Harvard name did not suffer was to resign my role at United Fruit." It was difficult to do, Cabot said, because he believed in United Fruit but he said he also felt that it was "a good thing to do for Harvard." Cabot suggested that this was the right pathway for Howard: to resign as dean of the School of Public Health thus sparing Bok the need to make a decision and, at the same time, ensuring that the negative publicity would go away. Cabot said that after he had resigned from United Fruit he felt better and suggested that should Howard follow that path that he would "feel much better" for having done so.

Howard had no intention of resigning. He listened to Cabot respectfully but gave no hint of what his plans were. The idea that he would resign from the deanship for doing what he had been charged with accomplishing by Bok struck him as preposterous, but he was always decorous, and his decorum held during this luncheon meeting. Howard admits to little in the way of resentment toward Cabot, but it is important to set the context in this case because the truth for many generations was that Harvard was very much a class-based institution. Certainly it was a university that pursued intellectual excellence, but it was also a college where the sons of the most socially prominent families from major cities in the United States and Europe were welcomed. Others—whether Jews, immigrants, the poor, or blacks—were unwelcome. When Howard was rejected by Harvard initially, Thomas Cabot was serving within the Cabot Corporation, a global mining company founded by his ancestors. Cabot was a member of one of the university's elite social clubs as well as a member of a half dozen or more exclusive social and country clubs in the Boston areas. On vacations, Cabot explored the wilds of northern New England, even writing a book at one point about the best places to paddle a canoe. The issue of class that hung over this particular lunch meeting was mentioned by neither man and, perhaps, noticed by only one of them, at least consciously.

The summer progressed slowly and painfully for Howard. He did not understand why Bok was taking longer than a week or so to render his decision in the matter. From Howard's point of view, he had done everything that Bok had asked, and more. He had gone into a stale, underperforming institution with a tenured faculty strongly clinging to the status quo and he had made significant changes that, in Bok's view and in the view of many others, had significantly improved the school of public health. And if Mr. Cabot didn't want Howard to create a splash at fair Harvard, there was no way that Howard could possibly do what president Bok had asked him to do *without* creating a splash. But now, as June wore on into a steamy July, Howard found himself largely avoided by senior faculty members as Bok silently considered the matter.

Letters poured into Bok's office in support of Howard. John C. Bailer III, MD, PhD, a visiting professor of biostatistics, wrote to Bok that he was "very deeply troubled" by the faculty's treatment of Howard, adding that "I believe that the Dean is correct on every significant point." Peter Braun, MD, clinical director at the Center for the Analyses of Health Practices, wrote to Bok that "I believe that Dean Hiatt was appointed with a strong mandate for change, in particular with a charge to project the School of Public Health more forcefully into the quest for answers to the underlying health problems of populations, to the teaching of key professionals in the field, and to the pursuit of studies which would help solve some important current problems of health nationally and internationally. I believe that Dean Hiatt has set forth with great vigor to achieve these ambitious goals." Maurice S. Fox, professor of biology at MIT, wrote to Bok that he had spent a sabbatical year at the School of Public Health under Howard's deanship and found "new and exciting directions apparent at the school." David G. Freiman, MD, professor of pathology at Harvard Medical School and pathologist in chief at Beth Israel Hospital, wrote to Bok that Howard's initiatives at the School of Public Health were "imaginative and appropriate." Irving H. Goldberg, Harvard Medical School professor of pharmacology and chairman of the department, wrote to Bok that "It is with incredulity that I recently learned of charges brought by certain members of the senior faculty at the School of public health against" Howard. Letters of support came from UCLA, the Roche Institute of Molecular Biology, the Esther A. and Joseph Klingenstein Fund in New York, Columbia University, the Dana Farber Cancer Institute, and more. In addition to many letters sent to Bok, Howard also received many letters expressing support for him—from Hugh R. Butt, MD, at the Mayo Clinic; from Victor Cohn at the *Washington Post*; from Ivan Diamond, MD, PhD, associate professor at the University of California at San Francisco; from Alain Enthoven, professor of management at the Graduate School of Business at Stanford, and others.

Howard held a strategy meeting at his home at one point and asked Arnold to attend. "He was in command," Arnold recalls of the meeting. "He was making sure his flanks were covered. He brought together his loyalists, the people who liked Howard very much." And these people, in turn, reached out to other Harvard faculty members who went to Bok on Howard's behalf and made clear their support for him, reminding Bok of the portfolio for change that Bok himself had given Howard. Scientists, including Konrad Bloch, the Nobel laureate in physiology or medicine, argued to Bok that letting Howard go would be convey a message that there was no room for serious science at the School of Public Health.

Among those working in support of Howard was Don Berwick. "I remember when the faculty rebellion took shape, there was a meeting where [faculty members] called for his resignation," Berwick later recalled. "He went to a meeting and talked about his vision and stood up to these guys. I wonder if he himself, in retrospect, was a little too confrontational. I remember his being attacked by these backward thinking faculty.... I thought what he did at the moment seemed quite courageous."

The *Globe* article by Loretta McLaughlin noted that part of the conflict dated back to Howard's appointment in the first place and resentment among faculty that he did not possess a public health background. The fury of the protesting faculty members was contrasted within the article by descriptions of the course Howard had set at the school. The reporter noted that when he was originally appointed Howard "was expected to turn the public health school in new directions, particularly research and training in health systems management, health economics, and health policy decision making, based more solidly on business principles and practices."

The article noted that Howard had

> forged strong beginnings of programs aimed at training "new kinds of public health professionals" with expertise in other fields, such as law, economics, engineering, business, and social and environmental sciences. On both short and long-term bases, he has developed fellowship programs for journalists, government officials, legislative assistants, health planners and those generally involved in influencing health policy. He also has enlarged faculty sharing with the Harvard School of Business Administration, the Radcliffe Institute, and Departments of Engineering and Economics.

While Howard believed Bok was taking too long to announce a decision, Bok felt he had little choice but to take the case made in the letter under advisement and take the time necessary to examine it. When the dissident faculty members presented him with the petition to fire Howard, Bok said "I felt I have to take this seriously, not that I have grave doubts of my own about Howard but it was important that I didn't just turn them down flat. That would have sent a message that the administration was not really interested in listening to the faculty and would have increased the level of resentment. I looked at it carefully, and talked to a lot people. I wanted them to feel that the process by which I arrived at this was something the faculty couldn't quarrel with."

It took until nearly summer's end for Bok to render a decision in the matter. On August 24, 1978, Bok told a meeting of the SPH faculty that Howard had his full support to continue as dean. In a page one article, the *Globe* reported that "Bok not only retained Hiatt as dean, but also declared 'my full support for the continued efforts of the dean to strengthen the school'"[1] The result of his deliberations, says Bok, was clear: "I delivered a very stern message," stating emphatic support for the changes Howard sought to make at the school. Bok recalled that some young faculty members came to him at the time; he recalls "Harvey Fineberg saying to me, 'wow, you set these people back on their heels.' After that the faculty knew that like it or not they were going to have to live with it." What was so striking about Bok's decision was summarized in the *Globe* article: "On every point raised by the dissident faculty, Bok replied the faculty's contentions were not supported by the facts. While noting that "the situation is tangled," Bok said he was "not persuaded by the specific complaints set forth."

Based on his training and experience, Bok was unusually well qualified to serve in judgment of this matter. He had received his law degree from Harvard and served on the Harvard law faculty as well as dean of the law school before becoming president. A deep familiarity with the workings of justice were in his bones. Was he biased because he had made the original appointment of Hiatt and only months earlier persuaded him to remain as dean? Certainly his instinctive preference would have been for Howard to remain, but his decision in the matter was far deeper and more thoughtful than mere reaction. In the two months he took to make his decision he held numerous meetings with the dissident faculty members. And he investigated. He looked carefully at the record and made his judgment based on the facts. The dissidents had charged that Howard had mismanaged the school's finances, but Bok rejected that, stating in a prepared statement, according to a *Globe* article, that Howard had been "following fiscal strategies that had also been used in other school units without creating 'inappropriate financial risks.'" Bok stated: "If anything could endanger the financial base of your faculty it would be continued public controversy of the kind that has preoccupied us this summer."

Complaints of ineptitude related to slow processes by the dissidents were easily turned aside by Bok, who said that delays reflect "a justifiable desire to hold out for appointments of the highest possible quality." Bok's wisdom was clear in his ruling: "The effort to make major changes in a school is always painful, threatening and divisive. In short, the situation is tailor-made for acrimony and conflict." Bok continued:

> There are grave dangers in seeking a change in leadership. Whether you choose to admit it or not, the resignation of the dean will be interpreted by many, many people as a victory for those who oppose substantial reform and a signal that continued change will be exceedingly difficult if not impossible.

The decision by Bok was nothing short of a devastating indictment of the dissident faculty. He found no merit whatsoever in any of the major complaints the dissidents had made. This was an embarrassing moment for this group of faculty members who, feeling threatened by change at the school, sought to pillory Howard. They wished to have the status quo continued. Howard was Bok's agent of change; they attacked him, and they were repudiated.

The entire affair was damaging to Howard—to his reputation and to his self-confidence. He had never before faced such a challenge, and "he didn't pick up the early signals," says Arnold Hiatt. The entire affair, says Arnold, was "very costly to Howard's self-esteem. It hurt him deeply." In his private memoir, Howard conceded that there were "things, looking back, that I might have handled better.... But I am not sure that there was any way to do what I was recruited to do there without blood on the floor. The committee appointed by President Bok to evaluate the school reported that they found entrenched mediocrity and systemic dysfunction."

Bill Hsiao, whom Howard had hired in 1974 and who believed Howard had accomplished nothing less than transforming public health education at an advanced level, says that Howard "paid a huge personal price" as a result of the controversy. "This was the first time a majority of senior faculty of a Harvard school had asked the president to remove a dean. It made headlines in the *New York Times*." And Hsiao saw the toll it took on Howard. Though he remained a strong supporter of Howard's, Hsiao questioned whether Howard had the chance to develop the full range of capabilities needed to lead such a complex organization through such rapid and extensive changes.

"Howard had the vision to transform the school but Howard did not know how to lead a complex organization through change—to change a complex organization. He was trained as a medical doctor and he also was a very good laboratory researcher. As chief of medicine at Beth Israel he was leading doctors but not managing a diverse group of people. He did not have to deal with the financial people, with nurses, or unions. He is a very amiable and friendly person but to lead a complex organization with different people in different disciplines who have different perspectives and where each department is trying to protect its interests and power is difficult—Howard did not know how to deal with these power centers."

Perhaps what ultimately mattered more than anything else to Howard was the continuing evolution of the school into something quite different from what it had been when he took over; into something that was very much aligned with Howard's vision of where to take the school. Under the leadership of subsequent deans—including Harvey Fineberg, his immediate successor—the school continued to grow stronger. "It is not, strictly speaking, accurate to say power is the only way to change an academic institution," he wrote in his memoir. "A second way is time: Bring in new faces and new ideas so that they will be ready when the passage of time thins out the implacable resistance. That is what happened at the Harvard School of Public Health. It is now a very different place, as President Bok acknowledged in his letter to me written ... eight years after I had departed."

The Bok letter was warm, and handwritten over a number of pages. While a crucial affirmation for Howard of the good he had done at the school, it came years later than, in his view, it should have. This, even in his tenth decade, was deeply upsetting to Howard. He felt that he had gone into one of the most troubled schools in the university, taken on a faculty determined to protect the status quo, and done so at Bok's behest. That Bok had come to Howard on the eve of his planned departure for Yale Medical School and asked him to stay was an indication of Howard's willingness to fight one of the toughest battles of Bok's presidency. "How much would the warmth and generosity of that letter have meant had it come when I was the beleaguered dean and in need of encouragement from outside!" Howard wrote in his memoir.

> Indeed, those times were so trying that if I had known what lay ahead, I honestly think I would not have taken the job, not without some serious guarantees of help from the president instead of vague, general promises. There is no question but that, going in, I was naïve about what would be required—for example, that to do what I had in mind I would need to hire new faculty with areas of expertise that were unrepresented at the School of Public Health, and that would cost money, lots of money that the school did not have and that its alumni were not, for the most part, in a position to contribute. Had I been aware, I would have insisted upon certain conditions at the outset.
>
> Perhaps this is the best I can offer in the way of lessons learned: Do the homework. Do not stint on your "due diligence." I had less than a week from the time I was offered the job at the School of Public Health before I had to tell the President

of Yale whether I would come to New Haven to be dean of his medical school. I accepted that short lead time, and my decision process suffered from the lack of a thorough exploration that more time would have afforded. I had rejected earlier offers of medical school deanships, at Johns Hopkins and Columbia, after extensive investigation led me to believe that conditions necessary to accomplish what I intended could not be achieved. I think it likely that a less hasty exploration of the situation and personnel at the Harvard School of Public Health would have led me to the same decision.

In an interview in early 2016, Bok was highly complementary toward Howard's performance as dean. "I think he really did turn that school around," said Bok. He said that changes made under Howard's leadership made the School of Public Health a really solid part of the university. The foundation was laid by Howard and had he not done that it would have been very, very hard because mediocrity would have been entrenched and difficult for anyone else to deal with. Howard had the difficult task of making changes in an adversarial atmosphere that enabled the School of Public Health to improve not only while he was dean but also in the years after he had left the school. Harvey Fineberg, Howard's successor, said Bok "was able to capitalize on what had been done under Howard and none of that would have been possible without what Howard was willing to do at considerable personal expense." "When I left the presidency [in 1991]," Bok noted, "the school of public health was really flourishing." Bok recalls spending a day at the school in the company of the six other members of the Harvard Corporation after Howard had completed the task of remaking the school "and the excitement was really palpable. There were good people in charge of the departments involved with problems in the world of major importance and there was a lot of excitement among the Corporation members with what they were doing. It was a totally different atmosphere then. Everything Harvey [Fineberg] did built upon the really heavy and often unpleasant lifting Howard accomplished."

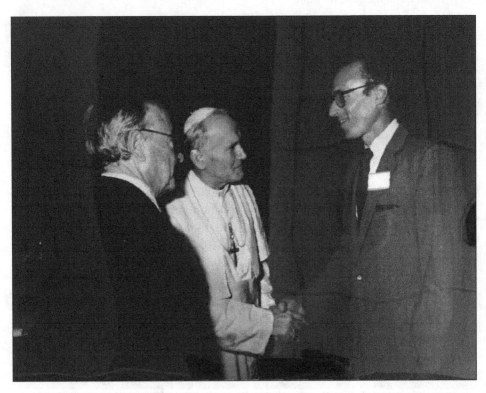

Figure 6.1
Howard Hiatt meeting with Pope John Paul II, December 1981.

6 Shifting the Post-Putsch Focus to a Larger Stage

Half of the tenured faculty had lobbied for his resignation, but after Bok had rendered his decision, Howard was still there. Most astonishing to him was the fact that, of the faculty members who had signed a letter that said, among other things, that they could not continue to work with him as dean, not one left the school. In his memoir, Howard wrote, "I had waited anxiously through the summer for Derek's decision, apprehensive lest he ask me to leave. But when the decision came, I realized it was only slightly better than the outcome I had dreaded. For, of course, I had to return to the School."

The obvious question is, why? Why, having been vindicated, did he not simply turn his back on the whole sorry situation? The answer was the same reason for which he had acquiesced in Derek's refusal to accept his resignation the year before: he could not walk out on the people he had brought to the school, especially the young people just beginning their careers, among them Milt Weinstein, Don Berwick, Bill Stason, and Harvey Fineberg at CAHP; the Fellows under Don Hornig at IPH; the new greatly expanded biostatistics department, now under the leadership of Marvin Zelen and already considered by many the leading department in the field. Nor could he leave Fred Mosteller, who had agreed to extend his time at HSPH beyond what he originally promised and assumed the chair of the unsteady Department of Health Policy and Management. As he saw it, he had been appointed to do a job; he had recruited people to help him carry it out; but the job was only partially completed. The president of the university had affirmed his support for what he had been recruited to do, and he could not leave.

Besides, there were still things he intended to do at the school. Funding was going to be a continuing problem, with many fundraising efforts blocked by the faculty unrest. But there was one very positive development in that respect. A relationship with the Harvard Business School had grown from the Executive Programs in Health Policy and Management. When John McArthur became dean of the Business School, he told Howard, "Your graduates are not going to be able to support your school—they don't make any money. My graduates do not have that problem. I am going to introduce you to a couple of them and suggest that they might want to get to know the School of Public Health." One result was a continuing relationship with an HBS graduate who was then CEO of Rohm and Haas, a chemical company in Philadelphia. He was an important supporter of cancer prevention work at the school and subsequently endowed a professorship of cancer prevention.

As chair of the Department of Biostatistics at HSPH, Fred Mosteller had "made Biostatistics into one of the School's crowning jewels," observed Howard. "The positive implications of having Fred Mosteller at the School of Public Health cannot be overstated. He made its biostatistics department into one that ranked with the statistics departments of any university in the world." Mosteller had also proved a crucial leader of the new Department of Health Policy and Management, when he took over as chair. So now, with Mosteller firmly at the helm, the Department of Health Policy and Management soon became a base for work in areas ranging from healthcare costs to quality of care to the need to make medical services more widely available to impoverished people.

One of Howard's goals as dean was to establish teaching programs in the quantitative analytic sciences that he believed were urgently needed by physicians at teaching hospitals and others who needed to carry out clinical research. He had earlier focused on the School of Public Health as a potential platform for introducing such sciences (biostatistics, statistics, epidemiology, and, later, decision sciences) into medical education. Now he tried to expand the training available at the school for clinical investigators to do research on the outcomes of diagnostic and treatment programs involving hospitalized and ambulatory patients and population groups. This was the foundation for "evidence-based medicine," that is, medicine that avoids diagnostic procedures and treatments for which evidence of positive outcomes is lacking in favor of those that have been demonstrated to be effective. This could improve clinical care by showing which tests and treatments were likely to work, as well as reduce costs by eliminating tests and treatments that had no positive benefit.

The principal teaching program of the school (and of all schools of public health) was the MPH, or Master's in Public Health, and this would serve as the vehicle for such an undertaking. The traditional MPH program was used to train physicians who wanted to serve in municipal departments of public health, at the Centers for Disease Control and Prevention, or to address the health problems of people in developing countries. To construct an MPH program for clinical researchers would require not only faculty from the School of Public Health, but also clinicians who understood the clinical problems for which better decision tools were needed. Howard was confident that he could readily enlist the clinical collaborators he needed from the teaching hospitals of Harvard Medical School. He recruited a young physician who came to the school and consulted at length with senior faculty about adding to the MPH program this kind of quantitative and policy training.

But opposition was widespread among the senior people at the school, and among many of the junior people, too. In a vote at a faculty meeting, the proposal to add to the MPH program was overwhelmingly defeated. It wasn't until much later, when Howard had left the deanship and gone to Brigham and Women's Hospital, that he helped develop what was called the Clinical Effectiveness Program. Later, after much pleading by SPH officials, Howard agreed to "return" it to the school (from Harvard Medical School, where he had developed it) as an MPH curriculum. It subsequently became the largest of the MPH programs and the school's biggest revenue-producing program.

Opposition and resistance came in many forms. One particular instance of that resistance served as a constant reminder to Howard that attention must be given continuously to keeping up with the cutting edge of whatever discipline future deans or chiefs will be dealing with. When Howard arrived at the school his attention was drawn by Lewis Thomas, then the head of the school's visiting committee and president of Memorial Sloan-Kettering Hospital in New York, to Myron ("Max") Essex, a scientist in the microbiology department at the school. Max had been at Sloan-Kettering, and Lew was familiar with his work on the cat leukemia virus. Thomas told Howard that he considered the work important. Further, he said, Max was valuable because he appeared to be the only member of the faculty at the school with a background in molecular biology.

Four years later Max came to Howard's office to tell him that he was planning to leave because Roger Nichols, chair of microbiology, had told him he had no place in the department over the long term. Howard consulted

Thomas, who said he thought it would be a serious mistake to let Max go, not only because he was a promising young scientist, but also because it would be a signal to others that molecular biology had no place at the School of Public Health. Howard reported this to Nichols, who insisted. Cat leukemia, he said, had little significance for public health, and *he* was the head of the department and it was his view that Essex should not be kept. Howard reminded Nichols that a chair was an administrative position conferred by the dean, and if he as chair could not see his way to keeping a molecular biologist of scientific promise in his department, then Howard as dean would have to change the departmental leadership. At that point, Nichols resigned as chair, and the result was a furor at the school: "How dare the dean dismiss a department chair?"—with the subtext, "Which of us could be next?"

In 1986, Essex shared the Lasker Award with Robert Gallo and Luc Montagnier for contributions in AIDS research. Essex's portion of the award was for showing, through his studies with cats, that retroviruses could cause immune suppression, and for detecting and characterizing the HIV protein now used worldwide for diagnosis and for maintaining the safety of blood for transfusion. For Howard there was a very important lesson here: the resistance of the chair of a microbiology department to new biological concepts that were spreading with excitement among serious scientists should stand as a warning for future institutional leadership.

Howard also pursued interests that went far beyond the School of Public Health. From the time he was a teenager Howard had a keen interest in public policy issues. In high school he followed events unfolding in the world closely enough to be able to host a weekly radio program in Worcester. During his army training before medical school he had reviewed the Associated Press wire each morning and announced the news highlights over a public address system to other soldiers at Fort Devens, Massachusetts.

By the 1980 presidential election the issue of nuclear war was under intense discussion throughout the United States and other parts of the world, and key participants within that debate were a number of Boston-based academics from Harvard, MIT, and other universities. A large number of them came together to lend academic weight to the antinuclear argument. During a symposium on the issue at Harvard in 1980, Howard delivered the main address to a gathering of hundreds of academics at the Harvard Science Center. This was no street protest of angry young people, but rather a measured discussion within a group where most were scientists, including many physicians. At the time, Ronald Reagan and George H. W. Bush, both candidates for president, had indicated that they considered a nuclear war survivable. The idea of the meeting, Howard wrote, was to counter this simplistic approach and "lay out in detail the effects of nuclear detonations on populations and infrastructure, in order to illustrate the obvious but seemingly ignored fact that after such an attack, medical services would be overwhelmed if not destroyed.... Because most of the surviving casualties of a nuclear attack would be burn victims, I obtained and incorporated a detailed account of the treatment of a badly burned young boy at the Shriners Hospital for Children, the burn unit at Mass General."

Anthony Lewis, a *New York Times* columnist (and long-time friend of Howard's), was in the audience that day and described the gathering as an "extraordinary two-day symposium on the medical consequences of nuclear weapons ... organized by Physicians for Social Responsibility and sponsored by Harvard and Tufts medical schools."[1]

Dr. Howard H. Hiatt, dean of the Harvard School of Public Health, spoke in measured medical terms about the effects of a single nuclear weapon on the Boston area. He drew on a respected study published in 1962 [by the *New England Journal of Medicine*]. It assumed a bomb equivalent to 20 million tons of TNT—a thousand times as powerful as the Hiroshima atom bomb but by no means the largest now in the armories.

That one weapon would destroy everything within four miles. The bomb crater itself would be half a mile in diameter and several hundred feet deep. Beyond the four-mile radius of total destruction a pressure wave, followed by winds of 1000 miles an hour, would build an enormous fire storm. Forty miles away, people looking in the direction of the explosion would be blinded by retinal burns.

Of the 3 million people living in the Boston metropolitan area, 2.2 million would be killed at once by the blast or fire storm. Of the survivors, Dr. Hiatt said, many "are badly burned, blinded, and otherwise seriously wounded. Many are disoriented. These are the short-term effects; the problem of radiation sickness will grow...."

Dr. Hiatt said all this in a quiet voice, and the audience listened in dead silence. Then he said: "The preparation of these remarks was for me a stressful experience. What purpose, I wondered initially, to describe such almost unthinkable conditions. But the conditions are not unthinkable. Rather, they are infrequently thought about."

By December of 1981, the nuclear issue had intensified on several fronts. Opposition to nuclear war among doctors was ratcheted up when the traditionally conservative American Medical Association overwhelmingly approved a resolution "to inform President Reagan and members of Congress about the 'medical consequences of nuclear war,'" according to the *New York Times*.[2] The article noted that "One of the most influential speakers and writers in the antinuclear arms movement is Dr. Howard Hiatt, Dean of the Harvard School of Public Health.

> Dr. Hiatt, who said he knew little about nuclear war except what he had read in the John Hersey book *Hiroshima*, recalls that he became interested after discussions with a colleague, Dr. John Burke, head of the burn care unit at Massachusetts General Hospital.
>
> Dr. Burke recounted his experience in treating a 20-year-old man who had been severely burned in an automobile explosion. The man needed 500 pints of blood, underwent six operations in which 85 percent of his body surface was covered with skin grafts and had to be kept on artificial respiration because his lungs had been scorched out.
>
> On the 33d day he died. Dr. Burke said the man reminded him of descriptions of victims of the Hiroshima bombing. Treating just that one patient had stretched the hospital's resources to the limits, and it is the only hospital in Boston with a burn care unit.
>
> Dr. Hiatt said he realized as he studied the issue that if the Russians dropped a hydrogen bomb on Boston, there would be half a million people dead and another half a million badly burned, and Massachusetts General would probably be destroyed. "When you have a problem that is untreatable and the costs are unbearable, you have to work on prevention," Dr. Hiatt explained. "Those people who talk about winning or surviving a nuclear war never considered the medical consequences."

The article reported that Howard had "devoted an increasing amount of time to talking about the dangers of nuclear war, including meetings in the last month with a group at the Vatican, with a seminar by the Mormon Church in Salt Lake City, and with Senator Paul Laxalt of Nevada, one of President Reagan's closest friends. Dr. Hiatt says he would welcome the opportunity to talk with Mr. Reagan. "I have the naive belief," he said, "that if I could just sit down and tell the President what happens to a burn victim, he would react like everyone else.'"

In December 1981, the nuclear arms issue attracted the deeper involvement of Pope John Paul II.[3] Howard was invited along with about twenty others to a meeting at the Vatican Academy of Sciences to discuss the nuclear issue. The other Americans invited along with Howard were Victor Weisskopf, a physicist at MIT who had been part of the atomic bomb development at Los Alamos; David Baltimore, biologist and Nobel laureate at MIT; and Marshall

Nirenberg, a biochemist at NIH, who had also won a Nobel Prize. The discussion, Howard wrote, centered on "what message would be appropriate to suggest to Pope John Paul.

> It was decided that it should focus on the medical implications of a nuclear exchange, and as one of the few medical people there, I played the major role in developing the message. Over two days we discussed and then drafted a statement, which we presented to the Pope. He met with us for several hours, thanked us warmly for the effort, and then asked us to carry it as his message to the heads of the four nuclear powers: Leonid Brezhnev, Margaret Thatcher, Francois Mitterand, and Ronald Reagan.

Two weeks after meeting with the pope, a four-person U.S. delegation met with President Reagan on December 17, 1981. In his memoir, Howard vividly recalled the event. When Reagan greeted the delegation he remained standing, conveying his impatience with the session and requiring everyone else in the room to remain standing as well out of deference to the president. Howard recalled in his memoir:

> The meeting with Reagan began late in the day. He clearly did not welcome the occasion, but he had had no choice, since it was at the request of the Pope. He received the four of us plus the Papal Nuncio, the Pope's representative in Washington, in the Oval Office....
>
> Viki [Weisskopf] made introductory remarks and said that since there was important medical content in our message, the U.S. group had asked me as a physician to summarize the Pope's message. I began by referring to the treatment for the serious injury that the President had suffered earlier that year at the hand of the would-be assassin. I apologized for personalizing my message and said that I had no knowledge of his treatment other than what I had read in the newspapers, but it was my impression that the doctors and nurses at the George Washington University Hospital Emergency Services had saved his life. Unquestionably, the President answered. Had three or four people with similar medical needs been hospitalized at the same time, I went on, the resources of the Emergency Services could not have coped. Any number above, perhaps, two would have had to be sent to other institutions. Again, the President agreed quickly with that proposition.
>
> Then I told him that estimates prepared by our own Defense Department made it clear that if a single nuclear weapon exploded over Washington, there would likely be several hundred thousand people in the President's condition. George Washington Hospital would no longer exist, nor would other hospitals or indeed any buildings within a radius of miles. I was concentrating on what I was saying and paying little attention to how the President looked, but Viki reported to me later that he blanched at that point and began to speak of Armageddon.

The *Crimson* reported that after the White House meeting Howard said that Reagan "acknowledged ... that a nuclear exchange would end civilization as we know it and that it is impossible to reconcile this with thoughts that one can win or survive a nuclear war." The *New York Times* reported that "The four scientists are not sure what effect they had on Mr. Reagan. But Dr. Howard H. Hiatt, dean of the Harvard School of Public Health and one of the papal delegates, said he believed that the President 'surely listened and acknowledged what we said.'"[4] The article continued:

> Dr. Hiatt, who has concentrated on the medical consequences of a nuclear attack, said he described to Mr. Reagan what would happen if a one-megaton bomb was exploded over Washington. "I told him there would be 800,000 people in shock from burns and radiation.... Given these facts, those people who talk about winning or surviving a nuclear war don't understand what they are talking about."

Howard's work on the nuclear issue led him to further study on U.S. defense spending. This was a classic liberal-conservative tug-of-war. Taking the position that the United States should spend less money on defense was a natural ideological extension of Howard's antinuclear work. Anthony Lewis of the *New York Times* wrote a column in October 1982 that focused on a commentary article Howard had written in the *New England Journal of Medicine* in which, as Lewis writes, Howard

> calls on doctors to make the public aware of what higher military spending may cost us in terms of health.
>
> The Reagan Administration's plan to spend $1.6 trillion on defense in the next five years requires a massive reallocation of resources, Dr. Hiatt says. It will necessarily reduce funding for other purposes, including health. And that will have concrete effects in the amount of illness and its cost to the nation.
>
> Immunization programs, as an example, may save in treatment of disease as much as 10 times what they cost. But cuts in Federal funds for 1982 will reduce the number of American children who can be immunized under those funds from 6.3 to 4.2 million. Dr. Hiatt also mentions cuts in money for venereal disease, lead-poisoning prevention and other programs.
>
> Then there is research. The research budget of the Defense Department has been increased 26 percent, Dr. Hiatt says, while that of the National Center for Health Services Research has been cut 45 percent. The cuts in fundamental biological and health research, he says, "will adversely affect the health of our own generation and of future generations."
>
> He also mentions nutrition programs, which have been severely cut—$1.46 billion slashed from Federal child nutrition programs, for one. The medical damage

resulting from malnutrition or disease in early childhood may never be repaired, and may be immensely expensive to society.

"Americans," Dr. Hiatt writes, "might reasonably compare the 'savings' on such health programs with the $4.5 billion allocated this year for the MX [missle] program; the $100 million cost for each of the 100 projected B-1 bombers ... and the $4.2 billion requested over the next seven years for civil defense."

Dr. Hiatt makes a point of saying that he respects the expertise of military strategists in their field. But wise political decisions, he argues, require listening to advice from experts in many different fields and balancing the needs. His presentation of the impact on health is thus in a sense a metaphor for the adverse impact that steeply rising military expenditure will have in many areas.[5]

Among Howard's many friends at the university was James Vorenberg, who had become dean of the law school in 1981. Like Howard, Jim Vorenberg was an immensely intelligent man with a strong set of impressive accomplishments. A graduate of Harvard Law School, he had served as president of the law review and clerked for Supreme Court Justice Felix Frankfurter in 1953 and 1954. In the summer of 1972 he had served in a senior position on the staff of Watergate special prosecutor Archibald Cox.

In the late 1970s and into the 1980s, millions of Americans were filing malpractice suits seeking financial compensation for injuries suffered in hospitals and physician offices. This malpractice crisis as it was known was evidenced by increasing numbers of law suits, and sharply rising malpractice insurance premiums for many physicians. To Howard, this was exactly the type of issue that could benefit by a joint initiative between the disciplines of law and public health. Soon after Vorenberg became the law school dean in 1981, Howard proposed that they team up and tackle the issue of medical practice injuries. This collaboration would result in the Harvard Medical Practice Study, a research report that would prove foundational to the study of error in medicine for decades to come. Malpractice was a significant area of concern for individual physicians and leaders of hospitals and physician groups as well as the general public.

Jim recommended that Howard connect with Paul Weiler from the law school faculty. Working with Weiler, Howard defined the scope of the project as "a study of the medical, legal, and economic consequences of medical injury." This was an enormous undertaking, and to get some form to the project Howard and Weiler decided to initiate an in-depth study in one state. Their strong preference was to focus the work within Massachusetts and Howard had high hopes this would occur. He placed a phone call to the president of the Massachusetts Medical Society for the crucial permission to access Massachusetts hospital records. To his surprise, the woman began by saying, "I know you. You saved my life." She turned out to be a woman Howard had met at a cocktail party five years earlier. Met is an understatement. In fact, at the party the woman was choking and Howard performed the Heimlich maneuver, quite likely saving the woman's life. That, however, was not enough to persuade her to endorse the study in Massachusetts. For a variety of reasons, she said the timing was not right. She said that she thought doctors were viewed somewhat negatively at the time and that the proposed project could make matters worse.

But a doctor who had been at Harvard Medical School while Howard served on the faculty heard about the malpractice study and contacted Howard. The physician, David Axelrod, was serving as health commissioner for the state of New York and was thus in an ideal position to advance the study. Axelrod told Howard that the malpractice issue was of great interest to New York governor Mario Cuomo. He said, "Governor Cuomo has asked me to prepare legislation to address the malpractice crisis. In looking at the medical and legal literature, all I find is anecdote. If you can carry out the study that has been described to me, it would provide me with the basis for proposing the legislation that the Governor wants." New York would provide access to hospital records for the study.

Since it would be all but impossible to gather information on all medical injuries in the state, Howard saw the need to identify a statistically valid sample. He enlisted the help of Nan Laird, chair of the biostatistics department at HSPH and a protégée of Fred Mosteller, to help with this critical part of the work. He recruited a number of other physicians including Troyen Brennan, a lawyer and a doctor, with both an MD and a JD. They calculated that the study would cost about $3 million. Howard went to Axelrod with this proposal and Axelrod, in turn, brought Howard in to see Governor Cuomo. "I apologized to the Governor for the size of the budget. 'Doctor,' he said, 'our physicians are now spending $1 billion a year on malpractice insurance, which actually means the people in the state of New York are spending that money. If for $3 million you can provide us with information that will spare us those costs, I will consider it a great bargain.' Never before or since have I had a research project funded so readily."

The support of Axelrod and the governor gave Howard and his colleagues "access to the entire record of hospitalizations in New York State for the year 1984" and the team then dug into the records of a random sample of hospitals throughout the state of New York provided by Nan Laird. Gathering those records and identifying patterns was an enormous undertaking. Howard recruited Lucian Leape, a former Boston surgeon who had just completed a year studying health policy at RAND in California, and invited him to join the study team. Howard had to work to persuade Leape to join. "I said I was not really interested—that I didn't want to study malpractice," Leape recalled. "He said it was much broader than that—that we were trying to understand who gets injured and how, what the costs were, etc. That began to sound interesting."

Job one was to define what constituted negligence. This was critical because the study was designed to look at one kind of medical error, preventable (negligent) error. So what, exactly, was a *preventable medical error*? There was no generally agreed upon definition in the literature. In his memoir, Howard defined it this way:

> To clarify the distinction between negligent and non-negligent injury, think of two patients hospitalized for serious streptococcal infection. Each is given penicillin, and each has a severe reaction that leads to kidney damage requiring additional weeks of hospitalization. These injuries were caused not by the problem that led to hospitalization but by the treatment, but only one was the result of negligence. The first patient had never received penicillin before, and therefore there was no way of predicting that she would react as she did. Her medical injury was not the result of negligence. The second patient had reacted badly to penicillin on an earlier occasion, so the information that she was sensitive to it was available and should have been accessed, whether through her records or by questioning her or her family. Her medical injury was negligent.

With the definition in mind, the team went into the field, "to train doctors to gather information," according to the book *The Best Practice*,[6] "Leape and Brennan would travel across the state running training sessions in the evenings for local doctors who would actually conduct the work of reviewing records. Over the course of most of 1989, Leape, Brennan and colleagues studied the records of more than 30,000 randomly selected patients who had been discharged in 1984 from 51 randomly selected hospitals throughout the state. It was the largest study of its kind ever conducted."

The findings of the study were stunning: Of the 30,000 patient records studied 3.7 percent "of patients suffered an avoidable injury that prolonged their hospital stay or resulted in measurable disability." Some of these injuries were fatal. Projected nation-wide, it amounted to 100,000 preventable deaths a year in American hospitals. The significance of the research was obvious, and the *New York Times* reported the news on its front page on January 29, 1990, calling it "perhaps the most comprehensive" study of malpractice ever undertaken in the United States.[7] The story noted that the study found that "thousands of hospital deaths and tens of thousands of injuries are tied to negligence each year but that relatively few victims seek recourse in the courts." The *Times* article continued:

> The Harvard professors, who come from the university's medical school, law school and school of public health, supervised a review of the records of 30,195 randomly selected patients who were treated in 1984 at 51 hospitals around the state.
>
> Teams of two doctors reviewed each hospital case to determine whether a patient suffered an "adverse event" or a "negligent adverse event."
>
> An adverse event was defined as an injury due to medical management that resulted in a prolonged hospital stay or reduced function at the time of discharge, like an unexpected infection or a fall from a hospital bed. The adverse event became negligent if caused by a failure to meet standards reasonably expected of the average doctor. Among such adverse events are careless surgery, misdiagnosis of condition, or improper prescription of drugs....
>
> The researchers conceded in the article that "judgments of causation and negligence are often not clear cut." To determine negligence, they established a scale of one to six points, with one being no evidence of negligence and six being virtually certain evidence. Cases were considered negligent if the ratings given by the two reviewing doctors averaged four points or more.

The Harvard Medical Practice Study was a landmark moment in modern American medical history. Its greatest revelation, of course, one that would endure for decades, was the foundational evidence that preventable medical errors were common and profoundly harmful in the United States. The study also revealed that the vast majority of patients harmed by a preventable medical error did not sue the hospital or physician. About one in seven patients harmed filed suit. It was clear to Howard and the team that most patients harmed received no compensation at all and that the legal system was an extremely inefficient pathway for patients to recover payment for the harm they suffered. The study, which analyzed the cases of 31,429 patients at fifty-one hospitals, found that eight times more patients suffered an injury because of medical negligence than filed malpractice claims and that sixteen times as many suffered negligence than received compensation through litigation.

Dr. Axelrod moved swiftly after the study's results were in to work with Governor Cuomo to propose "a system of no-fault medical malpractice insurance, which would compensate victims of medical injury without a judicial finding of negligence."[8] Axelrod said that many more victims of medical harm would receive compensation under the no-fault approach and would protect doctors from ever-increasing malpractice insurance premiums. The system would operate in a manner similar to workers' compensation: Patients harmed by a medical error would file a claim with an independent state board.

It was one thing for the study to be talked about in Albany by political leaders and reported in the *New York Times*. To physicians and other researchers, however, it was an order of magnitude more significant that the study was reported in a peer-reviewed article in the *New England Journal of Medicine*[9] (February 7, 1991). The study changed the trajectory of American medicine in that it led the way for additional research into the extent of medical error in the United States. The culture of medicine for many years had classified mistakes by doctors and other hospital and clinic staff members as "complications." Few doctors or hospital administrators believed that preventable errors in medicine were a real problem. The Harvard Medical Practice Study was a critical step in altering that belief.

After the study was published, Lucian Leape continued research on his own and, later, with others, eventually establishing the Lucian Leape Institute at the national Patient Safety Foundation. Howard's friend and mentee, Don Berwick, also continued working on the issue and Berwick and Leape would later be among the key players in a landmark report from the Institute of Medicine, *To Err Is Human: Building a Safer Health System*, published in 1999. The IOM report found that as many as 98,000 Americans died annually from medical errors, almost exactly the same number indicated by the Harvard study.

The authors concluded that the best way to deal with medical errors was for physicians to immediately "investigate them to understand their causes. You don't need to be a psychologist to realize that people won't report and won't discuss errors when you punish them for it. So, the focus on [mistakes by individual doctors] has a perverse effect: Not only does it not prevent most errors—It prevents us from knowing about them!"

Sadly, the proposed no-fault legislation in New York never progressed. Its chief proponent, Dr. Axelrod, suffered a debilitating stroke just months after the study was completed and never recovered. But in a remarkable turn of events, *To Err Is Human* became the most widely distributed report the IOM ever published and it launched a national movement to better understand and prevent medical errors.

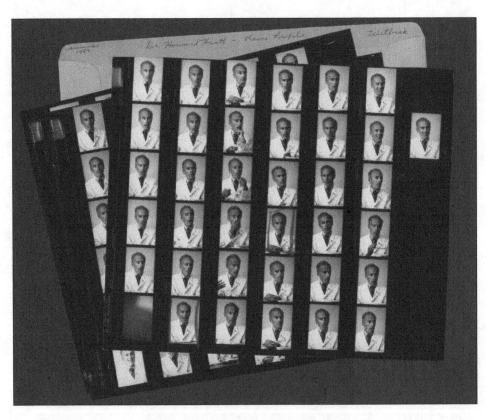

Figure 7.1
Contact sheet of Howard Hiatt once again in white physician's coat at Brigham and Womens Hospital. (Photograph by David Whitbeck.)

7 Taking Flight Again with Clinical Effectiveness Tools to Improve Health and Healthcare in America

As unpleasant as his experience as dean of the School of Public Health had been, the truth was that Howard had accomplished a great deal. He had, in fact, modernized the school in the way he had set out to do. He had brought in new faculty and new energy, and he infused the school with greater rigor in a number of departments. The fact that he was reviled by a number of senior faculty members bothered Howard. He had, throughout his life, managed to get along with people fairly easily. This was the first time in his life that he had faced anything remotely like the level of enmity expressed by the faculty.

Like most people who seek to achieve at a high level in their lives, Howard was nourished by positive feedback, but that had been in short supply during his SPH years. He did receive a handwritten letter from Derek Bok: "I cannot begin to describe how much better SPH is in every way from what it was in 1971," he began. "There is a sense of excitement, of student enthusiasm, of high faculty morale that is quite palpable. All this, as we both know, could not have occurred without the enormous effort you devoted to shaking the faculty out of its complacency and lifting its aspirations and its standards.... [Accomplishments in the future] will depend crucially on the progress you made against immense forces of inertia and convention." Howard was very pleased indeed with the letter, but would have welcomed it a good deal more had he received it in 1984 as he was departing the SPH. "I realize," Bok concluded, "how lonely and difficult your efforts were and how at several points you might have wished for stronger, more immediate support from my office. At this point, however, when one can assess the results objectively after the elapse of several years, the verdict seems clear, and you should feel extremely proud. For my part, I am simply extremely grateful." As it was, however, Bok sent him the letter seven years later, in 1991.

Howard began to wind down from his role at SPH in 1983 as he prepared to depart in 1984. His dozen years as dean were, mercifully, coming to a close. Bok thought it was time for a change at the school and Howard certainly felt it was time for him to do something else. He was fifty-eight years old and he was completing the least pleasant professional engagement of his life.

> I ended my days at the School of Public Health quite depressed. Although—or perhaps because—I had achieved a great deal of what was on my agenda, the stance of most of the senior faculty continued to be negative. The School was vastly different from what it was when I arrived, but getting acceptance for further changes I wanted to initiate continued to require a great deal of pressure on my part—not, for me, a pleasant way to proceed.

The constant tension and conflict, the unceasing opposition to Howard's ideas among much of the faculty, had made, he reflected, for a "bruising" experience. "When, in 1984, I stepped down from the deanship I must confess that I felt battered." Howard was convinced as he left the deanship that his "reputation in the greater medical world had been seriously compromised by the turbulence at the School. I feared that the message was 'Hiatt causes trouble he can't handle, and clearly he has little interest in medicine anymore.' Many of the professional colleagues with whom I had had close relations during my days at Beth Israel Hospital and Harvard Medical School were no longer very close. Most still wondered why I had given up medicine for public health and either hadn't followed what I had done at the School or were not in a position to evaluate it."

Never in his life had Howard faced a situation where he was at such a loss professionally. He was unsure what to do next; uncertain where to turn. He described this period in his memoir as "a striking contrast to the days when, as chair of medicine, I had been accustomed to receiving prestigious offers." But now he found himself with one job offer on the table, an opportunity from the Kaiser Family Foundation to lead that organization. "I had little interest in the idea of running a foundation, and" was not at all "enthusiastic about moving to California."

He needed a break and he took one in the form of a one-year sabbatical to work on a book about the challenges within the U.S. healthcare system. He headed to Washington to work on the book under the auspices of the Institute of Medicine. For the second half of the sabbatical year Howard was located at the King's Fund, a London think tank. It had been years since Howard had last been in London as a researcher for a year and the experience of being back in that city and connecting with old friends lifted his spirits. At the same time, he was making good progress on his book.

More and more, Howard was thinking about the challenging and flawed nature of the American healthcare system and he was excited to be exploring some of the most difficult issues in his book. Part of the reason he sought to spend the second half of his sabbatical in London was that he knew from his earlier time in London that the British health system, despite obvious flaws, generally provided excellent care to the great majority of the population.

The sabbatical year was crucial to begin to slowly help restore Howard's sense of confidence. He had been beaten down at HSPH and so too had his reputation. It hurt him deeply. He had become dean of HSPH based on a personal appeal from the president of Harvard. This came as he was being offered immensely prestigious positions at Johns Hopkins and Yale and being invited to discuss such possibilities elsewhere. He was much in demand. After he left the School of Public Health, much of that demand evaporated. "After HSPH I was no longer in demand anywhere except where people knew me," he lamented.

His spirits were as low as they had ever been in his professional life. But there was something deeply meaningful in the many friends Howard had made throughout his career. While the bitter taste of his experience with a group of dissidents at the school of public health was still in his mouth, the reality was that throughout his career prior to HSPH he had enjoyed excellent relationships with scores of physicians and other professionals and even at the school he had many supporters who greatly respected him as a professional and admired him as a person. And it was from the ranks of these many past colleagues and admirers that hands were extended to him.

One of those people to reach out to Howard was Dr. Richard Nesson, who had been Howard's deputy at Beth Israel Hospital. Now, in 1984, Nesson was president of Brigham and Women's Hospital, one of the most prestigious medical centers in the world, and Eugene Braunwald, another colleague of Howard's, was now chief of medicine at the Brigham. Nesson and Braunwald reached out to Howard and urged him to join them at the Brigham "as professor of medicine and senior physician with carte blanche to create my own portfolio." This offer came at exactly the right moment and helped restore, to some extent, Howard's belief that his reputation in the rarefied world of academic medicine had not been entirely tarnished. Though he had no clear idea of what he might do in such a position, he readily accepted the offer from Nesson and Braunwald.

"For Dick to offer me a place at the Brigham was the first example of a kind of reversal I have been lucky enough to experience more than once in my professional life—when a protégé becomes the leader, a mentee the mentor," Howard wrote in his memoir.

Howard was pleased to be at the Brigham but the truth was he really didn't have a clear idea of what he was going to do. That, however, changed quickly when Howard saw an opportunity to teach and mentor more intensely than he had ever been able to. And while this may have been unconscious, it was a chance to turn away from changing institutions to changing individuals, something that must have seemed at that point in time so much more appealing. He believed that he had been fortunate to have had some wonderful mentors and when he had a chance to select a whole team of smart young physician researchers to head his divisions at Beth Israel, he took great delight in mentoring them all. They, in turn, were grateful for his time, attention, and caring and when he left Beth Israel they gave their chief a framed photograph with each of their signed photographs and an expression of their admiration and gratitude. This picture hung in his office at the School of Public Health and it went with him to the Brigham.

At the Brigham, Howard's growing interest in teaching and mentoring developed along two lines: global health and clinical effectiveness. Howard's interest in global health grew deeper at the Brigham. His interest in engaging in public dialogue and global health emerged in various forms including public speaking and writing. In another op-ed article in the *New York Times*, Howard wrote:

> Of the 28 million people in Africa with AIDS, no more than 25,000 have access to medications. Officials of both Western nations and some affected countries— like South Africa, which has millions in immediate need of treatment—have said that poor countries have too few clinics and doctors and that their populations are too poorly educated to allow treatment of all infected people. This contention has become familiar in the debate over international financing to treat H.I.V.
>
> But it is a misconception. At a health center in Haiti, a country at the very bottom of the economic heap, H.I.V. infections are controlled as effectively as in America. And the success at this health center, sponsored by Partners in Health, a nonprofit charity affiliated with Harvard Medical School, could be replicated all over the world if the wealthy nations chose to provide the financing. The barrier

to the use of AIDS drugs for all H.I.V. patients is not some physical or educational impossibility; it is lack of will.

The center is in Cange, an impoverished village of small houses with corrugated roofs and dirt floors. There and nearby, care is delivered with skill and personal attention comparable to that in American teaching hospitals.

The compound was begun in 1983 by Paul Farmer, a physician and anthropologist now at Harvard Medical School, and the Rev. Fritz Lafontant, a Haitian Episcopal priest. Working with Dr. Farmer and Jim Yong Kim, another American physician-anthropologist, are Haitian doctors and nurses and about 200 community health workers, who make this model of health care succeed.

About 1,400 of the patients have H.I.V.; of these, 100 of the sickest receive the advanced medicines used to treat AIDS in the United States and now function normally. Their care is supervised by the local health workers, who are trained at the clinic. The health center's operations are financed by donations, and the doctors will treat another 100 desperately ill patients with the AIDS drugs if they can persuade drug companies to donate them.

Partners in Health also applies the principles used in Cange at a center in Peru and one in Mexico. In each case, training community health workers allows the development of a system that can offer sustained treatment for people ill with hard-to-cure diseases. The center in Lima has cured more than 80 percent of patients with drug-resistant tuberculosis—something many tuberculosis experts and even the World Health Organization had thought impossible.

What these doctors do to treat H.I.V. infection is a small effort against a huge worldwide problem. But they have shown that if we do not treat the millions of Africans who are dying of AIDS, it is because we have chosen not to, not because we can't.[1]

Howard generally received excellent feedback on his articles. He enjoyed writing these short pieces but he also for some time had wanted to put more of his thoughts and learnings together in a book. After leaving the School of Public Health Howard devoted considerable time to this venture and to writing his book, *America's Health in the Balance: Choice or Change?* published by Harper & Row. The seriousness and timeliness of the topic, along with the fact that the book was written by someone of Howard's standing, earned a review in the *New York Times*. The paper's lead reviewer, Christopher Lehmann-Haupt, wrote:

Few informed readers need to be reminded of the bleak state of affairs that prompted Dr. Howard H. Hiatt to write this drearily titled yet important book. The United States is potentially the healthiest country in the world, yet by the standard measurements of life expectancy and infant mortality we are relatively sick, and we are paying more and more for what inadequate medical care we get.

What is new about *America's Health in the Balance* is that Dr. Hiatt believes that steps can be taken to cure the patient. Drawing on his experience as clinician, research scientist, teacher, administrator and student of other countries' medical systems, he offers a diagnosis and a procedure for healing.

What sums up his argument most concisely is Garrett Hardin's famous 1968 essay on overpopulation, "The Tragedy of the Commons." In it the author showed how separate farmers, reasonably assuming that an additional grazing cow or two will serve their interests and do no harm to a public pasture, will nevertheless, as an aggregate, ultimately achieve the destruction of those grounds through over-grazing. "Freedom in a commons," Mr. Hardin concluded, "brings ruin to all."

Dr. Hiatt cites Hardin's essay in connection with the mass application of such expensive medical procedures as coronary bypass surgery, but by implication the analogy applies to the larger point of his book. Individual American doctors, rightly assuming an obligation to avail their patients of the best health care possible, are as an aggregate pushing our medical resources beyond their limits. The result is rationing by default.

Moreover, unlike the farmers in "The Tragedy of the Commons," American doctors and their patients do not have equal access to the commons. Too many specialists, for example, take up more than their share of space; while the poor and elderly, among others, are shut out. The further result is inefficient allocation of both cost and care.

What Dr. Hiatt poses as a solution is to take the best of the health care systems of Britain, which, he believes, produces better results than ours; of Canada, which has succeeded since 1971 in controlling costs and at the same time providing universal access to medical services, and of China, which despite its continuing third-world status, has since 1949 achieved the health standards of an industrially developed nation.

Roughly what his proposals boil down to is to guarantee universal access to the commons, but to build a fence around it with gates kept by general practitioners, and to appoint a committee to decide how the land within would be allocated. For instance, such a "God committee," as the author sometimes refers to it, might decide that no one over a certain age would be entitled to, say, a kidney transplant. He calls the resulting system Health 2000 and imagines how it could be running by the turn of the century.

Obviously, Dr. Hiatt is much more specific than this summary suggests. Indeed, he illustrates each step of his argument using actual, albeit pseudonymous, case histories, which are easy to identify with and therefore compelling to read. He surveys the latest developments in medical high technology, managing simultaneously to impress us with their wonders and to make us realize the impracticality of their mass application.

He is positively decorous in conveying the same message that Ivan Illich expressed more bluntly about a decade ago in a book called *Medical Nemesis* (a work that Dr. Hiatt surprisingly leaves off his extensive bibliography): one of the problems with medicine in America is that nobody wants to accept the inevitability of death. In short, for a book on such a depressing subject, *America's Health in the Balance* is surprisingly engaging.

Still, it leaves one wondering how Dr. Hiatt's complex, if practical, proposals are going to be implemented. Rachel Carson's *Silent Spring* it is not, nor Betty Friedan's *Feminine Mystique*, nor even Jonathan Schell's *Fate of the Earth*—all books that to some degree or other captured the public's imagination. One can only hope that committees are already sitting, ready to consider to Dr. Hiatt's recommendations. Perhaps a few powerful citizens will pay attention. Maybe a politician or two.

Meanwhile, one feels vulnerable to certain frustrations. Take the matter of smoking, for example. Dr. Hiatt points out somewhat hopefully that awareness among Americans is growing "that cigarette smoking is responsible for one third of all fatal cancers and one quarter of all deaths." He suggests that a committee in charge of health priorities would achieve enormous economies simply by abolishing the noxious habit of cigarette smoking. Fair enough. But considering the deeply ingrained history of tobacco in America, you have to wonder: can America's health really be cured by anything as pragmatic as Dr. Hiatt's committees?[2]

Ironically, when Howard submitted his manuscript to Harper & Row, he suggested that the book be titled *Medical Lifeboat—Will There Be Room for You in the Healthcare System?* Unfortunately, his editor at the publishing house rejected that title in favor of *America's Health in the Balance*, which the *Times* reviewer termed "drearily titled." The paperback edition however carried the title that Howard had initially suggested.

The book was fairly widely and well reviewed, but it did not achieve the goals Howard had set for it. He had hoped it would be the kind of insightful call-to-arms that would make for a best-seller and influence the direction of change and innovation in U.S. healthcare. Howard lamented that the book fell short of the goal with a melancholy observation in his memoir: "My mother and a few of her friends were favorably impressed by the book, but it didn't prove to be the best seller that might have led to important benefits to America's healthcare system."

In fact, the book was viewed as important enough to receive an additional review, albeit rather brief, in a *New York Times* health column: Health care in the United States is already rationed, Howard Hiatt argues; the country urgently needs a fairer apportioning of resources that will never be limitless. Those whose bills are paid with the help of private or Government health insurance get more than their share, he contends, while more than 35 million Americans - one-third of them children -are left to scramble for medical attention. "Jumbled policies and blinkered initiatives are literally killing many of us," Dr. Hiatt insists in this clear and persuasive book. The United States spends $450 billion a year on health, but ranks 17th among nations in low infant mortality, 16th in life expectancy. Dr. Hiatt, a professor of medicine at Harvard University Medical School and its School of Public Health, prescribes health insurance for all. He suggests regional control, as in Canada, perhaps by state agencies. Everyone would have a doctor who is a general practitioner, as in Britain - where people live slightly longer than Americans and most physicians get along without six-figure incomes. He is candid about British deficiencies, notably long waits for nonemergency services, and the fact that "many fewer Britons with kidney failure between fifty and sixty-five years of age, and almost none over that age, are begun on dialysis." But he says choices are unavoidable. A universal health system, Dr. Hiatt maintains, could reduce wasteful practices, such as unnecessary surgery and superfluous visits to specialists. His priorities for redirecting the resulting savings include improving community care for the poor, home care for the elderly, preventive medicine, research and medical scholarships.[3]

Howard didn't just write about improving health and healthcare in the United States; he worked for many years to find and implement ways to make it both more efficient and equitable. A couple of decades before he arrived at the Brigham, when he was chief of medicine at Beth Israel Hospital, Howard had been keenly interested in finding ways to integrate analytical sciences into clinical work. He saw clearly that the use of statistics, biostatistics, and epidemiology could help advance patient care by identifying best practices. His pursuit of evidence-based medicine drove him in this direction. He discussed this with his friend Cyrus Levinthal, a biologist on the faculty at MIT, and they decided to make a significant move in this area. But the timing proved off. Before they could get anything going Levinthal accepted a position as chair of the biology department at Columbia University.

"By the time I left Beth Israel, research in clinical departments in hospitals had been profoundly changed by the revolution in biology that enabled researchers to focus at the molecular level on how the causes and treatments of medical problems could be better addressed. But there had been no comparable change in the methods for assessing the effectiveness of different methods of treatment, whether new or existing."

Howard raised this issue in an article in the *New England Journal of Medicine* in 1977. His view was that many common procedures in medicine had been done countless times without sufficient evidence that they actually worked. There had long been too much reliance on anecdote in medicine,

Howard believed. But the time had come for a shift to more scientifically based evidence. Howard had pushed to make measurement and analytics more important throughout HSPH while dean there and now, at the Brigham, he believed it was time to create a program in clinical effectiveness to educate doctors about measurement sciences. Very few physicians knew even the basics about measurement sciences. The mathematical sciences were very much needed in medical training, in Howard's view, but were largely absent. Young doctors learned the healing techniques from older, more experienced physicians in a way that was similar to the apprenticeship process that had existed in Europe and elsewhere for centuries. The need was not only to equip doctors with the ability to measure their work and determine best practices, but also to analyze the value of care they delivered in economic and financial terms. This was an important issue in the 1990s as healthcare costs throughout the nation were rising rapidly and would become an even more urgent concern years later when the share of GDP going to healthcare reached an astonishing 18 percent, more than double the share of any other industrialized nation in the world.

One factor in particular that motivated Howard on the measurement front was the bitter experience he had had at HSPH. As dean, he had succeeded in increasing the amount of measurement science in public health courses and this was an important step forward. But he had sought to alter the Master in Public Health degree to make analytic science a more central part of the curriculum. As dean, he considered the program insufficiently rigorous and lacking in some areas, including quantitative analytical sciences. He was interested in supplementing that with a program offering an MPH in clinical effectiveness, which might attract physicians or nurses who might have an interest in public health as part of their work within a department of medicine. When this idea was put to a vote of the SPH faculty it had been defeated by a wide margin. The faculty was speaking clearly: The status quo was not only acceptable but desirable and there was no need for any such revision to the MPH program. The failure of the program to be given even a chance to get off the ground was deeply disappointing to Howard, just one more shot from a bitter faculty.

At the Brigham, however, he found enthusiasm for the idea of making medical care more measurable. He was convinced that statistical evaluation was woefully lacking in care delivery and he was convinced that major leaps forward were possible in this area. He had been talking with colleagues for some years about what he described as "evaluative clinical sciences—statistics, epidemiology, decision analysis, cost-effectiveness analysis, economics, ethics, and computer science."

Quantitative analytic methods equip doctors with the tools they need to measure and by measuring they can identify defects in the system and improve a variety of elements including access, the patient experience of care, safety, and quality.

> I believed that if those topics were included in the clinical education of medical students—and of practicing physicians—the quality of medical care would be greatly improved. In time, people equipped with these skills in the clinic and in teaching would populate academic departments of medicine, to the benefit of individual patient care as well as national health policy.... In addition, it was likely that regular assessments of the cost-effectiveness of different interventions could have important benefits for health care reform.

He was ahead of his time with this thinking. In part, it was the research scientist in him, and also in part it was the public policy person. He had delivered an important examination of American healthcare in his book and he could clearly see the need for more rigorous analysis of what worked and what did not. His instinctive belief was that many traditional approaches to care costing tens of millions of dollars annually had never been proven to be effective. He was focused intensively on evidence-based medicine a decade at least before it became a popular watchword throughout the world of healthcare.

At the Brigham, Howard engaged in a series of animated conversations on this topic with Lee Goldman, a cardiologist. Goldman was the perfect partner for Howard on this topic, for he was not only a cardiologist but also had significant experience in statistics. He was experienced at measuring healthcare effectiveness. These discussions were particularly exciting to Howard. He had just recently returned from his sabbatical and approached his undefined role at the Brigham with some anxiety, but the more he talked with Goldman the clearer it became that such a program was sorely needed within the medical center.

> We began with seven weeks of intensive work in the summer of 1985. We recruited three post-doctoral fellows in cardiology whom we knew and were able to persuade that the program would be interesting and that it would help them follow in the footsteps of mentors such as Lee Goldman. Their enthusiasm for

the study spread in the Brigham, and in the summer of 1986 we had eight participants. Most of these were graduates of a Brigham residency program and post-doctoral fellows in one of several specialties—cardiology, infectious diseases, endocrinology and gynecology—whom the first graduates persuaded to try the program.

The program covered seven weeks of intensive work in the first summer. All students took biostatistics and epidemiology and then selected two other courses from among economics, decision science, ethics and a few others. Those students who sought an MPH degree chose a research topic to work on during the rest of the year when they were back in their home departments. They worked in collaboration with two mentors, one from the PCE program faculty and one from their home department. They returned to the School for a second summer of seven weeks of course work, after which they were awarded an MPH degree by the Harvard School of Public Health.

The demand for spaces in the program demonstrated the hunger on the part of many physicians to learn about analytics and measurement. In the early years most of those joining the program were fellows at the four Harvard teaching hospitals in Boston, but very quickly word spread about the value of the course and that brought fellows and faculty members from universities throughout the country and later, the world.

After a few years, the program was so successful that "the School of Public Health agreed to incorporate a degree in Clinical Effectiveness in its MPH program." A few years later the MPH in clinical effectiveness would become "the largest single part of the School's MPH programs." By 2015 about 175 students were enrolled in the clinical effectiveness summer program.

The Clinical Effectiveness Program grew into one of the most academically and financially important parts of SPH. In 2016 it was described by the school as being "designed for physician-clinicians, fellows and faculty, who are seeking quantitative and analytic skills needed for clinical research or are interested in healthcare administration."

There have traditionally been many more applicants for the seats in the program than capacity. Thus, recommendations from senior faculty are required of all applicants and all participants must have completed their residency (or be in a residency program of longer than three years). The program includes two courses that last the full summer and constitute the program's foundation: biostatistics and clinical epidemiology. In addition, students have a wide choice of two half-summer electives that include medical informatics, linear and longitudinal regression, and improvement in quality in healthcare.

The program is intense and requires that all students remain "free of all clinical responsibilities during the seven-week period." Nine in ten students taking the course in the summer of 2015 were satisfied or very satisfied with the program. The magnanimity with which Howard decided to send the program back to be housed at the School of Public Health was characteristic of his generosity of spirit.

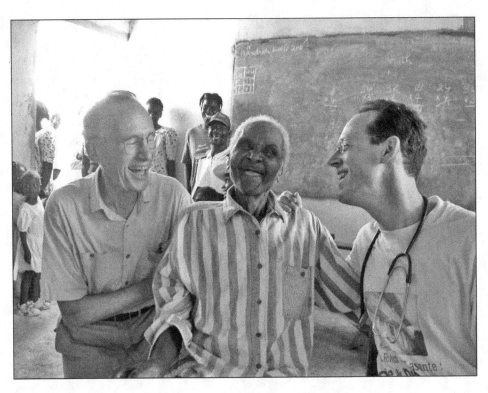

Figure 8.1
Howard and Paul Farmer laughing with a 104-year-old man in Haiti, 2004. (Photograph by Mark Rosenberg.)

It was this same generosity of spirit that turned Howard into an extraordinary mentor. Dr. Marshall Wolf was at Brigham and Women's Hospital in 1972 when Howard was appointed dean of the school of public health. Wolf was delighted to see Howard take the position because it meant he would no longer be leading Wolf's rival department of medicine at Beth Israel Hospital. At the time, Wolf led the Brigham residency program. Traditionally, Mass General Hospital had been the only serious rival for the Brigham in attracting the top residents, but under Howard, that had changed. "At Beth Israel Howard recruited a bunch of wonderful young people to run various divisions and that gave us at the Brigham a hard run for our money as the most attractive training program," recalls Wolf. Wolf did not know Howard particularly well but that changed when Howard arrived at the Brigham and began digging into the issue of global health. Like Howard, Wolf also provided guidance to Paul Farmer and Jim Kim.

Wolf had established a program that suited the needs and desires of Farmer and Kim perfectly. Back in 1972, Wolf and Dr. Gene Braunwald, Brigham's chief of medicine, set up a residency program for people who had done research while they were in medical school and wanted to maintain their research momentum. Under this program, residents would come to the Brigham as a pair. One would be in the hospital doing clinical training while the other would be in the lab conducting research. Over a period of three years each resident would do twenty-four months of medicine and twelve months of research. It meant four years of training—a year of internship and three of residency—instead of three, but physicians also pursuing a research track jumped at the opportunity. It was this program that made it possible for Farmer and Kim to share a residency, enabling the two men to train at the Brigham while at the same time working on their initiatives in

Haiti and Peru. And it was Marshall Wolf who introduced Farmer and Kim to Howard when Howard came to the Brigham. Marshall let it be known that he sent "all the difficult residents to talk to Howard." And Paul remembers that Marshall used to say "anybody who didn't have a very clear plan for their life, go see Howard."

Farmer had met and roomed with Jim Kim at Harvard Medical School, and there they realized they shared a passion for applying their skills to cure the world's poor. They would talk late into the night about equity and healthcare as a human right. In 1987, while still in medical school, Farmer, who had already had years of experience working with a clinic in Haiti, cofounded Partners in Health (PIH) along with Ophelia Dahl, Todd McCormack, and Thomas J. White. Farmer already had years of experience working with a clinic in Haiti. Kim, who had also worked in Haiti, joined Partners in Health as another cofounder months later.

By the time they arrived at the Brigham for their residency, they had already opened a clinic in Cange, part of the central plateau in rural Haiti, and were committed to spending time there. During the 1990s, Farmer and Kim together performed something of a medical miracle in an impoverished neighborhood in Peru. Farmer and Kim had a friend from Boston, a Catholic priest, who had gone to work in Carabayllo, a hot and dusty slum on the outskirts of Lima where he contracted TB. Though he came to Boston for treatment he could not be saved. When he died Farmer and Kim dug deeper into why the treatment had failed. They discovered that the priest had been afflicted with multidrug-resistant tuberculosis (MDR-TB), a deadly disease that spreads easily when not properly treated. This brought Farmer and Kim from Boston to Lima to research the situation. They found widespread MDR-TB within the Carabayllo shantytown. TB becomes drug resistant when patients take their medications irregularly or stop taking the drugs too soon, before all the tuberculosis bacilli have been killed, leaving behind some that are now resistant to that drug. It becomes multidrug resistant when this inadequate treatment occurs more than once. The bacilli that remain are now resistant to the first-line drugs and to the second and even third-line drugs. MDR-TB spreads rapidly, and—in a new patient—is often treated with the wrong drugs as providers presume the infection to be from a simple susceptible strain. Both Farmer and Kim knew that unless they could find a way to treat it in this resource-poor area many people would die. At the time, the course of treatment for MDR-TB was so difficult and expensive (estimated at $250,000 *per person*) that the WHO had issued a policy that called for *not* treating patients with the disease in poor countries. Without treatment, patients were left to die and to spread the disease further before they did. WHO leaders reasoned that precious finances could be used more effectively helping people suffering from conditions that could be treated at a reasonable cost. The lack of moral grounding of this policy deeply troubled Farmer and Kim. From their positions as staff physicians at Brigham and Women's Hospital, they initiated a program that performed the difficult task of, first, tracking down the right medicines at a price they could afford, and, second, caring for all residents of Carabayllo suffering from MDR-TB.

"Everybody in the medical world was absolutely convinced that you could not treat multidrug-resistant TB in a developing country," Kim explained during an interview. "The only experience was treating the disease in very highly specialized medical centers with access to very rare and expensive drugs with very highly trained specialists and all at a cost of $250,000 per patient! There was a lack of imagination because people had never been in a setting where there were lots of MDR-TB patients."

Farmer and Kim were able to spend a great deal of time in Lima during their residency because they had been able to work out a highly unusual arrangement with the Brigham. Dr. Marshall Wolf saw the passion and intelligence with which the two young physicians approached their work and he worked out an arrangement that allowed them to share a residency. It was a form of job sharing, except the job was being a physician in residence at a major hospital.

"Marshall allowed our research laboratory to be the rural health centers of Haiti," Farmer said. Farmer had majored in anthropology as an undergraduate at Duke. Even at that young age he was drawn to Haiti to try and understand the culture and to provide some kind of help to the people. He realized during one of his undergraduate trips there that becoming a doctor would enable him to provide hands-on medical help to many poor people.

As was the case at most hospitals, Brigham staff physicians were entitled to discounts on medications at the hospital pharmacy. Typically, doctors used this privilege to buy occasional medicines for family members. Farmer and Kim, however, had a different idea. They were purchasing large quantities of drugs for patients in Lima with tuberculosis and then transporting those medicines to Peru during their regular trips. No one within the hospital had paid any attention to this highly unusual activity until one day when the president of the Brigham confronted Howard and told him that "your protégés are in big trouble." While most physicians using the pharmacy for personal reasons charged $50 or $100 worth of drugs over the course of a year, it seemed that Farmer and Kim had run up a total of almost $100,000.

"They were taking the drugs and putting them in their suitcases and going to Lima and treating people," says Howard. "The president of the hospital said to me that Paul and Jim had been 'sweet talking the pharmacists out of these drugs each time they travelled to Peru.'"

Howard could not have been more thrilled! How wonderful these young men had earned MD and PhD degrees while at the same time somehow finding energy to travel to Haiti and Peru to take care of some of the poorest people on earth. The depth of their passion and commitment was magnificent and Howard felt a profound sense of joy being able to help them. He solved their immediate problem by placing a telephone call to a very generous philanthropist who promptly wrote a check to the Brigham for $94,000 to cover the full cost of the medicines. That money covered the cost of drugs that Farmer and Kim had already used and now Howard was determined to find a way to buy ever larger quantities of drugs for the patients in Lima.

Howard Hiatt went into his full helping mode. He had protected Farmer and Kim at the Brigham when their medications bill was revealed. He had helped them gain additional funding. And now that the results of the Lima work were in, he would help them spread the news worldwide. But WHO was a tough nut to crack. The TB staff there was resistant to the idea of treating multiple-drug-resistant TB because the medicines needed for this treatment were so very expensive. "The head of the WHO tuberculosis section at the time was Arata Kochi, a public health doctor from Japan who, it turned out, had been a student at the Harvard School of Public Health during my deanship," Howard wrote in his memoir. While Kochi had been a student, Howard and his wife had included him in a dinner at their home and Kochi had felt moved to be included. And he had never forgotten that dinner. When Howard asked for his help, Kochi's reply was, "anything you want, dean." Howard persuaded the American Academy of Arts and Sciences to host the meeting and obtained money from the Rockefeller Foundation to pay for it. Howard wrote in his memoir that

We invited fifteen or twenty tuberculosis authorities, as well as representatives from the Rockefeller Foundation, which put up the money for the meeting, held at the American Academy of Arts and Sciences in Cambridge. Paul and Jim presented their careful documentation of their results (85% cure rate in a poverty-stricken area), and the reactions were electrifying. On the spot Arata invited Paul and Jim to come to Geneva to present their results to a larger audience, and he insisted that I accompany them as well. At the larger meeting at WHO headquarters in Geneva there were over a hundred TB experts in public health from countries around the world, and the presentation created an equally strong response.... The WHO moved at once to change its recommendations to include a regimen for treating MDR-TB.

During their research into the challenges presented by MDR-TB, Jim Kim discovered that most of the drugs used to treat the disease were quite old and Howard, through his vast contacts, made arrangements for him and Kim to go to drug companies to try and convince them to provide generic versions of the medications. But because MDR-TB was not treated on a broad scale, pharmaceutical companies found little demand for the drugs and therefore didn't produce many of them. Howard brought Kim to a meeting he arranged with Gail Cassell, a contact of his at Lilly, the manufacturer of one of the key drugs needed to treat MDR-TB. After that Farmer and Kim were able to convince Eli Lilly Co. to let them purchase some of the medications—some of which were out of patent—at a reduced price for the purpose of their research project to demonstrate the effectiveness of proper treatment, and they arranged to purchase others from Chinese and Indian generic drug companies at a fraction of what the cost would have been in the United States.

Next, when Farmer and Kim were starting to get back very promising results from the first set of patients they were treating in Carabayllo, they hit another roadblock. They realized that these were just preliminary data and to get definitive results they would need to keep their treatment project going for another year. And this would require a million dollars, a million dollars that they did not have. Again, Howard came through. He told Jim and Paul to contact me, another mentee of his, at The Task Force for Child Survival and Development, a global health nonprofit in Atlanta. The Task Force had been started by Bill Foege, a physician-epidemiologist who had been the architect behind the eradication of smallpox. Foege was another mentor of mine and was now working closely with the newly established Bill and Melinda Gates Foundation.

Howard thought that through these connections—from Farmer and Kim to Hiatt to Rosenberg to Foege to Bill Gates—there was a chance of getting the million dollars that Farmer and Kim so badly needed to keep their project alive. I arranged for Paul and Jim to come to Atlanta and present their findings to Bill Foege, who was impressed by their vision, their passion and their commitment to the people who were suffering from MDR-TB. The core strength of The Task Force was organizing and sustaining the kind of effective coalitions that are needed to solve large-scale global health problems. I worked closely with Jim to put together an effective coalition that could continue their MDR-TB project, prove that their approach worked, change policy, and take this approach to scale.

In the course of putting this proposal together, we brought in new partners—the ministry of health of Peru, the Centers for Disease Control and Prevention, the World Health Organization, and The Task Force—and as we did this the cost of our proposal rose. When Bill Foege finally presented the proposal to Bill Gates, it was for a total of 44.5 million dollars. This was the largest TB program grant that the Gates Foundation—or any foundation for that matter—had ever made. And Bill Gates was nervous about giving this much money to a few people that he didn't know. Bill Foege was at the Gates Foundation headquarters when the funding decision was being made. Bill Foege had shown Bill Gates an article that Tracy Kidder had written about Paul Farmer for the New Yorker just a few months earlier, and in the article, Kidder mentioned that Paul had just one suit, and it was black so that when Paul had to clean the tip of his pen, he could wipe it on his pants without it leaving a mark. So when Bill Gates asked Foege "How do I know that this man Farmer is not going to take our 44 million dollars and go off and buy a very fancy car?" "You can be sure," Foege told him, "because anyone who has only one suit is not going to go off and buy an expensive car!"

That clinched it and this grant launched a seven-year program that showed MDR-TB could be treated effectively and cured in resource-poor settings. What made it possible to treat patients with a 90 percent success rate for less than $2,000 was the community health workers. These workers visited every person with MDR-TB every day and directly observed people taking their medicines. Even when there were side effects that made people feel worse, these community workers made sure patients took their pills every day. Every day, seven or eight medications for two years. Using community health workers made the program successful and led WHO to change their policy from one that said that when poor people in poor countries get MDR-TB they should just be left to die.

The new policy had at its core the principle of equity, a principle that Howard, Jim, and Paul had in their heart: whenever a person contracts TB, whether it be drug-sensitive or drug-resistant TB, whether rich or poor, regardless of where they live, they should be treated appropriately.

Howard remained totally committed to Farmer and Kim and never missed a chance to help. When the Division of Global Health was initially being started, Wolf says that Farmer and Kim were concerned about the amount of their time that might be required in the administration of the department. "They were somewhat uneasy about that," recalls Wolf. "They didn't want more administrative work and Howard stepped in and said I can help you do that. If Howard had not volunteered to help I am not sure there would be a division of global health."

Howard's presence in the division of global health—which continued beyond his ninety-second birthday—coupled with his years of administrative experience within the Harvard universe, meant that things ran smoothly right from the start and he provided Farmer and Kim with the support and freedom they needed to do their groundbreaking work. Their mission was to provide quality healthcare to the poorest people on earth. Since that time, they have become seminal figures inspiring caregivers in Haiti, Rwanda, Peru, Mexico, Russia, Kazakhstan, Malawi, Lesotho, and elsewhere. While Farmer has focused on curing the individual and the social circumstances that spawned the disease, Kim's focus has been on changing policy to cure the system. In early 2000, Kim played a central role devising and implementing an aggressive World Health Organization (WHO) program to treat AIDS in Africa. As a senior staff member at WHO, Kim recognized that those who worked in global health were effective at analyzing problems and proposing solutions and yet too often fell short when it came to implementing effective programs. When he returned to Harvard he founded the Global Health Delivery program to deal with this shortcoming. It was an important addition to the academic global health arsenal. Subsequently, he served as president of Dartmouth College and now leads the World Bank. Farmer has remained focused on his work as a physician at Partners in Health, at Harvard and Brigham and Women's Hospital in Boston, and in poor countries around the world. Farmer is one of the very small number of uniquely prestigious University professors at Harvard. Over the years, the two men have remained faithful in their individual ways to the mission they envisioned in their late-night sessions as young medical students, and grateful and still deeply connected to Howard.

At the time, the working definition of global health was anyplace outside the United States, particularly a place that was poor and underserved by traditional health resources. Once Howard had established a department of health policy and management at the school of public health, the idea caught on and spread to most of the U.S. schools of public health. This created a dichotomy: health systems of other countries were studied and taught through departments of global health, but the U.S. health system was taught and studied in departments of health policy and management. It was as if the United States were not part of the globe. In the minds of many politicians the United States had the best healthcare system in the world. But Howard knew otherwise. He had a broader view, developed in part, through his study of the British and U.S. healthcare systems, and he realized that while the United States provided the most expensive healthcare in the world, by almost any other measure it did not rank in the top twelve for the best quality of care and health outcomes. Howard thought the United States had a lot to learn from the other 200 countries in the world, especially from many low-income countries where, as Jim Kim put it so well, poverty encouraged innovation. Howard thought that the words *global health* should include health in the United States. And he mentored another physician who showed just how much the United States could benefit from lessons learned in the poorest of countries.

Heidi Behforouz was born in Iran to an American mother and Iranian father. Both of her parents were university professors in Iran, and when the Iranian revolution came, the family moved to the United States. As she grew up she developed a desire to find work that would enable her to address some of the social ills afflicting poor people. She chose medicine as her pathway. But by 1992, her second year at Harvard Medical School, she grew disenchanted. She was unable to see the connection between medicine and her desire to alleviate suffering among the poor and help achieve social justice. Nonetheless she graduated from medical school and then completed her residency in medicine at Brigham and Women's Hospital. During that period, she met Paul Farmer and Jim Kim. She told Paul that she felt she should travel back to Iran and care for poor people there.

"But Paul said, 'Don't go to Iran, come work with us,'" she recalls. "It was a godsend for me because I became part of a community of like-thinking people, which is what I had been missing." Thus was born a program she called PACT (Prevention and Access to Care and Treatment), a global health–inspired program aimed at bringing care into the homes of poor people in the Roxbury neighborhood of Boston. PACT was described by its leaders as based on a "model pioneered in rural Haiti" focused on "integrating community health workers (CHWs) [and global health principles] into primary care and mental health teams. PACT partners with clinics to develop the infrastructure, culture, quality improvement tools, and skills necessary to support effective CHW interventions for the most vulnerable patients." While still in medical school, Behforouz had visited patients at home in several large, subsidized public housing buildings. "There were many elderly people and people with HIV/AIDS, people with physical disabilities," she says. "What struck me was that people were dying in these buildings in this mecca of medical care, within walking distance of Harvard-affiliated hospitals. It didn't make any sense."

In 1997, Behforouz made her first trip to central Haiti, where she found that "the issue was that there was no healthcare. So PIH built an oasis of white stone and brought in not only medicine but doctors and food and schools." This facility provided ongoing care to persons with AIDS by dispatching community health workers to patients' homes to make sure they received and took their medications. But back in Boston—a city that prided itself on having the world's finest healthcare—this was not happening. Some people with AIDS received no care at all while others relied upon periodic visits to the emergency department. With support and encouragement from Howard, Behforouz and a team of community activists began visiting patients daily and directly observing them taking their medicines at home. Medication compliance soared and patients got healthier. The program improved health for patients while showcasing the effectiveness of CHWs. "These community health workers were people recruited from the community who spend a majority of their time in communities and homes," says Behforouz. "They bring to their work experience and understanding of the people they serve. They are a bridge between the community and institutions that have become so professionalized and siloed that it's hard to establish therapeutic relationships." A PACT program analysis indicated that the work by Behforouz and their teams significantly reduced usage of Brigham and Women's emergency department by PACT patients thus reducing Medicaid costs for these patients by an estimated 35 percent.

The work by Paul Farmer, Jim Kim, Heidi Behforouz, and others was rather extraordinary even for the kind of talented young doctors the Brigham attracted and trained and it was warmly embraced by the Brigham's chief of medicine, Dr. Victor Dzau, an accomplished cardiologist who had come to the Brigham from Stanford and who would go on to serve as chancellor at Duke University and president of the National Academy of Medicine. "Victor said to Paul and Jim and me that he thought there should be a residency in global health and that meant setting up a division of global health along similar lines to the department of cardiology or any other medical division." Dzau convened a meeting that included Farmer, Kim, Behforouz, and Howard. Dzau made it clear how excited he was about the work that was being done in places such as Haiti and Peru, and he had an idea for creating a new division at the Brigham that would be unique in American medicine. He proposed to start a division devoted to global health work, research, and study. It would be a division comparable in its scope and seriousness to the other major medical divisions such as cardiovascular medicine, and endocrinology.

Was such a division warranted? Howard noted in his memoir that many people asked that question assuming that "global health is simply another name for international health. Programs in international health have been numerous in schools of public health and also present in some medical schools. These programs have largely been concerned with studying diseases like malaria and schistosomiasis that are prevalent among people, especially poor people, living in tropical climates. Tuberculosis has been high on the list of diseases of concern to international health and, in recent years, HIV-AIDS has become one of the most serious international health challenges. But research on disease, important as it is, does not define the range of concerns of our group, nor is it what Victor had in mind when he proposed launching the new division. Rather, he recognized that what Paul and Jim had pioneered and what they and their young colleagues were practicing was a new way of delivering high quality medical care informed by the best research in areas where resources were scarce. Further, in part because of their anthropological training, they concerned themselves not only with disease, but also with the larger context of health issues facing poor people."

In his private memoir, Howard went back and interviewed Joel Katz, who had served as the original director of the residency program within this new division. Dr. Katz said the following:

> Graduating medical students in the early 2000's were increasingly interested in pursuing careers that focused on addressing health disparities, particularly those occurring in poor countries. Paul Farmer and Jim Kim's example inspired many such students to seek training at BWH. In 2000 or early 2001, Jim Kim and I met (at Pat's Place over cheese steaks!) to discuss how we could best serve such students' career interests, and at the same time start to formalize career pathways that would be recognized and rewarded—and result in clinical jobs—at teaching hospitals and medical schools. Jim suggested calling this a "Community Medicine Pathway" (which remains the label on the file that I started after that meeting and use to this day!), in recognition that populations in need were domestic as well as international. After review with Paul, we established criteria that training should be split between BWH and resource-poor settings (likely, but not required, to be PIH sites), residents would learn principles of program assessment/improvement and health advocacy, and residents would obtain an advanced degree (e.g., MPH) if desired. The detailed program design was delegated to a steering committee of Amy Judd, Margaret Paternek, Howard Hiatt and Joel Katz, as I recall, with many design contributions from Marshall Wolf, Joel Katz's predecessor as director of residents at BWH. Implementation required serial approval by the Department of Medicine (Victor Dzau), the Partners Educational Committee (PEC) and the American Board of Internal Medicine (ABIM).

In an interview a decade after the division was founded, Howard was asked by a reporter from the *Boston Globe:* "What made you say, this is something the hospital should embrace? There wasn't a model for a global health division at other academic medical centers." He replied: "You can't be exposed to Paul Farmer or Jim Kim and not think that this is the thing you should do. I was seduced by those two guys."

"Paul was the right person to lead the division and when it was raised with him he said, 'I will do it but we will call it global health equity.'" The phrase "global health equity" had first been coined and used by Bill Foege in 2000 when he was working with a team in the early days of the Bill and Melinda Gates Foundation to succinctly and clearly define their goal and mission. Paul and Jim worked closely with Bill Foege and admired him. "It was about fairness in access to health care for everyone. It was a recognition that health care is a human right." The name ultimately chosen for the division gives a clue to what it is about. What began as the Division of Social Medicine and Health Inequalities became, first, the Division of

Global Health, and then the Division of Global Health Equity. Equity means fairness. Thus, global health equity is fairness in access to quality healthcare for everyone. In the DGHE, this is a human right.

When you work with Paul and Partners in health you follow Paul's idea of liberation theology, it means a real commitment to helping poor people. It recognizes that if you want to do good you have to help the poor who have the least access and that to help the poor you have to *be with them*, to live among them, and to understand the conditions under which they live. When Partners in Health goes into a country to work, they do not visit and then return to the United States or some other rich country, but instead the PIH physicians and others live in the country among the poor people. This is a deeply compassionate approach to delivering care but it goes deeper than that. Compassion is "feeling with" the other person, feeling their pain and suffering, listening to them and identifying with them, but compassion by itself is not enough. Paul says that he has never met a poor person in a poor country who came to him and said, "what I really need is someone to feel with me." What is needed is *consequential compassion*, another phrase coined by Bill Foege, which includes action.

In practice that means doing what is necessary to make sure that poor people have equal access to the means of health—to diagnosis, treatments, nutrition, vaccines—to all of the preventive and clinical services that help a person achieve health.

In the fifteen years since the division was formed and the residency established, scores of physicians have successfully completed the program and gone on to do impressive work. In the process, it has established the Brigham as an international leader in global health. The combination of the division, the residency, and the close affiliation via Farmer between the Brigham and Partners in Health, has made the Brigham the go-to U.S. medical center for expertise in global health.

Howard had assisted in both setting up the department and managing a large part of it for many years, in no small part because equity and social justice had been the true north of his moral compass. Now the residency in global health equity was a way to extend his mentoring to a new generation of young physicians—even mentoring a new generation of mentors—and Howard took on the task of raising the funds to support it. Howard wrote about the division of global health equity in his memoir, telling only part of the story of how the residency got its name:

We knew that the creation of a residency in global health equity for young physicians was the most important step to be taken by the new division. Amy Judd, later the Division's administrator, called the residency the "feeder system" to develop leaders in the new field. But there were complications. The Brigham residency program, like those in every American teaching hospital, is supported by federal funding from Medicare, but this funding is restricted to programs that train physicians for medical care in the U.S. A residency in global health, directed at patients in other countries, must find its funding elsewhere. Therefore, we were going to have to do some serious fund-raising.

We began by seeking support for faculty for the new Division. My brother, Arnold, a businessman as well as my closest friend, and parenthetically one of the most generous and self-effacing people I know, has always been my best financial guide. It was to Arnie that I went to discuss this need. After first committing himself to give towards both the DGHE faculty and later the residency, he said he would also help us raise money. His first suggestion was, "See whether Frank Hatch might be interested."

At an earlier time, Arnie had asked me for some advice for Frank, one of his very close friends. Frank ran the John Merck Fund, which had been set up by the family that had founded the American branch of the Merck pharmaceutical company. Frank's wife Bambi was a Merck. Her brother John Merck had been severely impaired intellectually from birth and had a marked personality defect as well, which was referred to in the family as a "double disability." They had established the John Merck Fund, one of the missions of which was to address such combinations of neurological problems. In its early years, Merck awards had been used by a few medical schools to support departments of neurology or psychiatry, as well as for some specific activities in those departments. Frank was not satisfied with the results of these grants, and he was looking for advice. I told him that this was a particularly opportune time to focus on problems like the ones they were interested in, because research on the nervous system was moving forward quickly and with some very interesting outcomes. A whole new area of investigation, called neurobiology, was being built on this research and thus, funding young scientists who wanted to work in neurobiology would likely be very productive in discovering more about the kinds of brain dysfunction from which John suffered. After talking further with Frank and with Bambi, I recommended that the Fund invest in a program of fellowships for young neurobiologists early in their careers. I told them I thought that encouraging able young scientists to work in the field was the best route toward the kind of advances in scientific understanding they hoped for in the future.

Frank and Bambi accepted this advice. They set up the John Merck Scholars program and asked me to chair the committee that would select the scholars. I was able to assemble a stellar group to serve on the selection committee, including Molly Potter, Professor of Psychology at MIT; Torsten Weisel, then the President of Rockefeller University; and Eric Kandel, Professor of Neurobiology at Columbia. I directed the committee for more than fifteen years. Many important advances were made by the John Merck Scholars we selected, and when one of the first awardees (Linda Buck of the University of Washington) won the Nobel Prize in 2004, Frank Hatch and the Fund board were very pleased indeed.

During my time on the John Merck Scholars Committee, Frank and I had become good friends, so it was not difficult to approach him on behalf of the new division in global health equity. He told me at once that he liked the idea and said he would help raise money for it. He introduced me to other members of his family and several of his friends who he thought might also be interested. I then suggested to this group that the funds we raised for support of the first five years of the GHE faculty be named after Frank. Frank demurred. He said he would not welcome such an arrangement. Only after rather extensive discussions did he agree to permit his name to be used for the faculty endowment—with a condition. He would agree to the establishment of the Frank Hatch Scholars Fund if I would agree to have my name on the future residency program. I was no more eager than he to have my name used, though for a different reason. I saw the naming rights as an enticement for a serious donor who might endow the residency, and I was reluctant to give away the opportunity for free, as it were. In the end, I had to agree that my name could be used to solicit funds for the Doris and Howard Hiatt Residency in Global Health Equity in order to win Frank's acceptance of the Frank Hatch Scholars Fund, but I continue to be eager to give the name away in return for some substantial funding.

What Howard left out was that Frank Hatch wanted to have Doris and Howard Hiatt's name on the residency program because Doris and Howard had, in their push for global health equity, done so much for so many for so long. Howard continued:

> We invited Frank's relatives and friends to lunch at the downtown Harvard Club in Boston, and thanks to my brother's guidance and Frank's generosity, and to the affectionate regard in which Frank was held, it proved to be a successful fund-raiser. Among them, Frank's family and friends promised to fund an annual endowment of over $1 million to be used to support the first five years. We were ready to launch.

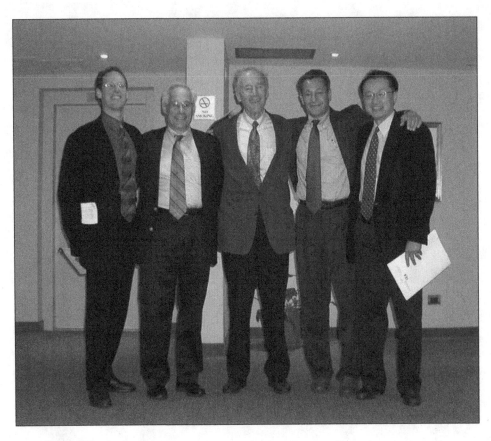

Figure 9.1
The Four Brothers. Howard with Paul Farmer, Don Berwick, Mark Rosenberg, and Jim Kim.

9 He Was Wholly There for Us

Howard was the leader who changed and improved two of Harvard's most important institutions—Beth Israel Hospital and the Harvard School of Public Health. He fostered the birth of the global health equity department at the Brigham. But the most important contributions Howard Hiatt made involved his role as a mentor, guiding and shaping the lives of some of the most influential men and women in healthcare. Through the decades he served as a counsellor, mentor, teacher, adviser, and friend to scores of young physicians, but perhaps his greatest influence as a mentor was his relationship with four Harvard Medical School graduates who became so close to one another—and to Howard—that they refer to themselves as "the brothers." Three of these four physicians—Don Berwick, Jim Yong Kim, and Paul Farmer—are among the most influential and accomplished healthcare leaders of their generation. I was lucky enough to be the fourth brother. Howard connected us and has been incredibly supportive of all of us. He has been very important in all of our lives. In late 2012 and early 2013, I sat down with each of my "brothers," and interviewed them about the role Howard has played in their lives. This chapter draws from those sessions.

Many of the young physicians Howard mentored were different. Most medical students were focused intensively on their education and training in medicine and gave little thought to broader political or public policy issues. But the four of us, while dutiful students in medical sciences, were also keenly interested in broader policy questions. Don Berwick and I, for example, not only took degrees from Harvard Medical School but also studied public policy at the Harvard Kennedy School. Paul Farmer started a clinic in rural Haiti while still a medical student and would go on to become an ambassador for health to the world. Jim Kim became interested in the broader policy question of how can the successes of the business world in actually delivering goods and services be applied to the work of public health, higher education and the elimination of poverty. Each of us was also different in that we had Howard Hiatt for a mentor. What follows are our personal reflections on how that came about and what it meant to us.

Don Berwick, MD

Howard is a gentle soul, but he is also exacting and professionally demanding of himself and those with whom he works. This was obvious at the SPH and many faculty members there reacted quite negatively to his demanding standards. Don Berwick, one of Howard's protégés and dearest friends, recalls the sting of Howard's criticism the first time they worked together.

> It goes back to a project I did at the Kennedy school when I did an MPP. I don't remember meeting him in any way other than causally before. Dick Neustadt was helping us to do work for a client. I took that on. The origin may have been that Howard approached Neustadt about the Northbridge project, the idea that HMS should take over an area of Boston—he called it Northbridge—so that the medical school could take over healthcare for that part of Boston. He wrote it up for the *NEJM*, and my assignment was to help him. So I met with him, he outlined the idea, and I went to work. My job was to interview people who might have opinions, like Rashi Fein, in the social medicine department, and John Knowles, then general director of Mass General Hospital. One of the people I interviewed was Leonard Cronkhite, CEO of Children's Hospital Medical Center. He was lukewarm about it, so when I wrote up the report, in my memo to Howard—and this was the Vietnam era, an anti-anything era, when I was approaching this with a chip on my shoulder—I thought how arrogant of Harvard, thinking it could fix anything. In that memorandum, I made what he thought was a big mistake. I said to Howard that one of the impediments was the animosity between you and Cronkhite, and that was a malapropism. What I meant was that there was a discrepancy. But I wrote down the word animosity. Within what felt like minutes, I was called to his office, and he was furious. He was shaking he was so angry. Did I know how much destruction I had done, how much damage could be done by leakage of this memo; he had nothing but the best of feelings toward Cronkhite. The fact that I didn't mean to say what I had said was irrelevant, he was just fit to be tied. I left shaken, then met with Neustadt, who told me I had really blown it—this was not how one talks to one's boss. That was a scary experience with Howard Hiatt. He left my life at that point and there was no contact with him for a long time.

Several years later, after Howard had become dean of SPH, he called Berwick, who was then a resident in pediatrics. Howard had found Don's class day speech quite thoughtful. During the speech, Don had "predicted that the SPH would go away and be merged into the Medical School. Howard knew that and said since you are about to do me out of the job, would I come over to meet with him." After they talked, Howard was very impressed with Don's energy and intellect and with his willingness to think a bit differently. He liked the fact that Don had completed the Kennedy School Masters in Public Policy program and he thought Don would be a good fit at SPH. He offered Don a job as assistant to the dean.

> My interactions with Howard were not extensive. And to be really honest I remember being frightened of him. My main insight was that he was an authority figure, and I remembered seeing him come down the corridor on the 10th floor and running the other way.

Howard played a decisive role at a pivotal moment in Berwick's career. Berwick was working on improving quality at the Harvard Community Health Plan and, toward that end, he was studying the work of W. Edwards Deming, the visionary advocate for spreading the lean methodology inherent in the Toyota Production System. Deming's teachings had been adopted by the Japanese automobile industry, which led to the transformation of quality in Japanese-made vehicles, radically altering the world of motor vehicle sales for good. Deming's thinking and methods had been applied throughout many manufacturing companies as well as in some service companies, but no one had ever applied his methods to healthcare. Berwick thought Deming's approach was an exciting way to improve quality and safety in care delivery and he shared his enthusiasm in a conversation with Howard. (This was 1988.) "I was telling him about the work of Deming and how excited I was, and he said, 'you must write this up. It has to be a *New England Journal* paper.' He was insistent."

For the next week Berwick immersed himself in the task. His paper, "Continuing Improvement in Health Care," was published in the *New England Journal of Medicine* in 1989. "It became the turning point paper of my career," says Berwick. "Howard caused that. I was just learning what would become the theoretical foundation of my work and to have someone of his stature come by and say this is worth pursuing. If he had not said that, I would not have written the paper, and I don't know what I would be doing right now."

When Berwick and several colleagues founded the Institute for Healthcare Improvement in Cambridge, Massachusetts, Howard helped procure foundation funding for a program of leadership development for health care professionals interested in the kind of improvement initiatives Berwick and IHI were promoting. "Thanks to Howard, for about a decade we always had about eight to ten young people, learning improvement," says Berwick, who notes that a number of those men and women have gone on to play major roles in improvement work in the United States, New Zealand, and the UK.

Berwick says that Howard influenced him in three important ways:

First, he is a source of encouragement; he is almost always saying "yes, you should do that." He is relentlessly affirming, immensely valuable for someone with my personality, raised by a father who was very critical, always brooding, always afraid something would go wrong, a very important antidote at every step of the way.

Second, through the introductions he has made. It is scary to think how many of the people in my life he is responsible for: Tom Pyle and Gordon Moore, he opened the door to foundations, the Commonwealth Fund and Frank Hatch. To put me in the same room as the people he has recruited. He is the world's greatest networker.

Third, not just for me, but modeling behavior, he is the person my whole family would model themselves on. He will always ask "How are the kids? Before we talk about me, let's talk about you." He is the model of civility, graciousness and caring. So, through these three ways: encouragement, connections, and by setting an example.

Paul Farmer, MD

I met Howard during my first year of medical school in 1984. He would always be there and was more than happy to just talk to us. He was the former dean of the School of Public Health and the urbane, sophisticated person who knew about social medicine. For many years, I didn't have an intimate friendship with him. Then Jim and I started at the Brigham in 1991, and he had an office on the Pike [the main hallway at the hospital]. Marshall Wolf used to tell anybody who didn't have a very clear plan for their life, "Go see Howard." And so see him we did, since Jim and I were the oddest ducks in the cohort, because our free time was spent in the field. Then we became close friends. I remember that by the time I wrote *Uses of Haiti* in 1994, I was so close to him that I would use his office, and brought the proofs of the book and put them in his office. I would just go by every day. When you have someone at the height of their powers and they make you believe that what you are doing is really important, especially if what you are doing is not fully embraced by mainstream academic medicine, it makes a real difference. You need people like that, especially to grow something new. You need protectors and mentors who are connecting you to a system that is full of resources. That's not why I went by and hung around with him. I did it because he was affectionate and kind and funny, with a wry, self-deprecating sense of humor. I felt like I had been "adopted" by Howard and his wife Doris.

Then an epidemic of MDR-TB was revealed to us in 1994–1995. Jim and I were making the transition that year to an infectious disease fellowship; we traveled between our field sites and the Brigham. Howard and Doris came to Lima. Between 1996 and 1997, I was really pushing hard, taking care of a lot of patients in Peru. It was a really difficult year; I got sick in 1997 with Hepatitis A. When we told Howard about the problems we were having with drugs, he asked, "Do you know Armen Tashjian? He was on the board of Eli Lilly." Howard intervened, and Jim went out there with him. We were trying to get these drugs, and I made Howard promise to turn his attention to the drug problems. They were available, but not being used. I used a little Catholic Jewish trick: wait until you are really sick and then make him promise. Then I went to France to recover. When I got back, feeling fine, Howard and Jim were deep in negotiations with the manufacturers. I said, "How is this going to get us what we need? We need lab capacity." Howard said that we should wait and see. Jim felt that policy change was important and would drag along the delivery science. He was right. We were working on the policy change.

Then in the fall of 1997, I spent a lot of time putting together a meeting of several experts. I knew the TB clinicians, Mike Iseman, Sir John Crofton, and all the Boston ones. I knew but had less favorable relations with the public health ones. So we used Howard to bring in those people from WHO. The clinicians were not so difficult. We feverishly prepared for the April 1998 meeting at AAAS. I was writing preliminary reports from the working group. By that time, Howard was in pretty deep. After the spring of 1998, Howard made a couple of trips to Geneva, Jim did too, then came DOTS-Plus and the Green Light Committee. Soon thereafter, we met with Bill Foege and you, at the Task Force in 1999. Then Howard and Doris came to Lima, which was when Howard suggested I should start a division dedicated to global health equity at the Brigham.

One more thing I would like Howard to acknowledge in his book: after we thanked him in 1998 for helping us get MDR drugs, he said this is good but don't think about asking me to do that for AIDS treatment. And that was just what we planned to do. Jim and I looked at each other with just that in our mind.

I very much wanted to go to Africa in 2003, but when Jim left for the World Health Organization, I spent a lot of time on the new division and Howie more than helped; he was vibrantly engaged in building it. I couldn't just cut off my connections and obligations to Haiti. Howie was the geographically present rock. The Gates grant helped a lot with that, helped to strengthen our position at Harvard and the Brigham. I didn't know much about that part of it.

It was 2008 when Jim went to Dartmouth as president of the college, so Howard again had to join me (not that he ever didn't join me). When Jim left, it was hard on us, because I had already started working in Africa, had moved my family there right before the 2010 earthquake in Haiti. I was named the division chief again when Jim left. Howard was the vice-chief, and we had almost twenty-five faculty. Jim had also been chair of the Department of Global Health and Social Medicine at Harvard Medical School. I had to apply to the dean for an assistant in an administrative position; it was out of a sense of obligation to the faculty. Now we have grown that department as well. Howard was always willing to step into administration medicine, willing to step in and be the central figure. I felt a little guilty but was not surprised. Other people might have been saying "I want to go live in a cave … or Falmouth," but he didn't do that. The earthquake aside; that was a huge disruption. But now both the Division and the Department are more stable and large. Jim and Howard's investments are protected. Howard always says you have to have someone ready to take your place. Now we have probably 120 faculty across the university. A large enterprise compared to other universities.

Howard has battered me with his affection over the years around a couple of key points: teaching, policy, and long-term legacy. I started teaching with Arthur Kleinman in 1986, so I had a lot of experience teaching and didn't have to be told. Looking back, Howard has won all those arguments. If your definition of leadership is developing platforms from which other people can lead, that is what I would like to do. I am trying to look forward to influencing the next generation of public health leaders. He made me look at that earlier and more recently. I didn't want to administer a department and now I administer two. I would have said I would rather do care in Haiti or Rwanda than teach Harvard med students, and now I teach *every* Harvard med student.

For my entire adult life—and I would rank my becoming an adult after starting med school when my father had just died—Howard has always been part of my life. Many of us are thinking that it would be a big mistake for Howie to totally retire. He loves mentoring students and entering into the chaos of other people's lives. And the recipients *love* it, too.

Jim Yong Kim, MD

I remember how intently and joyfully he listens to young people, he listens with great joy, and you can just tell he loves interacting with and trying to help young people. You can tell that he is a very wise man. There was a former Harvard Medical School dean who said to me that Howard Hiatt was one of the *enfant terribles* of the medical area; he was someone who didn't tolerate weakness or laxity in any program. I spoke to another person, a gastroenterologist, Benjamin Banks, an older doctor who had been at the BI and asked him "Do you remember Howard Hiatt?" He sure did; he told me he was so hard on me, he couldn't stand us old-time clinicians. *He wanted to know the evidence*. Dr. Banks remembered how hard-charging Howie was. I had almost the opposite memory: he was so impossibly dignified, polite, and thoughtful. He seemed to have money in the bank with so many people working on so many critical projects. I was blown away by his gentility. But he had been known as one of the most hard-charging physicians, with a commitment to excellence. He has an enormous bias for intelligent young people and when he decides you are worth investing in, he is behind you all the way. When he was young he could not tolerate mediocrity. I have come to learn that this is a good trait. Learning diplomacy is important, but an ability to sniff out mediocrity is even more important.

I first met Howie when one of the first projects we took on was to organize the MD-PhDs in the social sciences who were training at the Brigham. Howie wanted to do a seminar, my second year, 1991–1992. I had met him casually but started interacting more with him then. We wanted to get MD-PhDs in the social sciences to make presentations, and, I need to say, I failed miserably: only three people showed up at one of the events. I was miserable and Howie was clearly disappointed and I felt I never again wanted to have this experience of disappointing him so badly.

A few years later Paul Farmer got Hepatitis A and almost died. That's when we really started to work with Howie. We talked to him about getting MDR-TB drugs, and Howie really got involved calling people on our behalf and helping with our bills. He also arranged for us to have the MDR-TB meeting at the American Academy of Arts and Sciences in Cambridge, and he was also able to get Arata Kochi, who was then the head of TB at the World Health Organization, to come. That's when we saw how good it was to have him on our side.

The most memorable part of it was that he really did become my mentor right around that time. We had long talks about my future because I didn't see where my life or my career was going. I went to Peru thinking I would have the kind of relationship with Peru that Paul had with Haiti, but I found my focus would turn to the overall policy atmosphere and to the political economy of trying to make such a huge change in global health. I enjoyed seeing patients but I knew that being a clinician in poor countries was not how I wanted to spend my life. I actually felt badly about that. I felt that I *should* want to see patients all day but I was more interested in policy. Howie was the one who started encouraging me in this direction. You sit down with him and his face will light up and he is as thrilled to hear about your aspirations and achievements as your own parents would be. I hadn't ever seen that with anyone but my parents. He gave me the confidence to not follow exactly the path that Paul followed.

And that confidence was important because we were setting out to change the policies of huge organizations, like WHO and CDC, who said it was too expensive to treat poor people in resource-poor countries when they had multidrug-resistant TB. We also wanted to change the policy of USAID when they weren't ready to start treating people with both HIV and TB. Howie gave me the confidence and breadth of vision to go down that path. He took great delight in encouraging me and doing it in such a focused way. In those circumstances, you really need a mentor.

Every time I have made a change in my life—and this has been quite frequently—I didn't make a move without speaking to Howie. He was skeptical about my going to become president of Dartmouth; he wanted me to stay at Harvard and continue working with him and with Paul. He is one of the first people who found out about the World Bank opportunity [Kim is president of the World Bank] and his first reaction was total delight.

He has influenced me in so many ways but his greatest impact on me has been through a conversation we have been having over many years about what I should do with my life, as a leader. I wouldn't have done so many things without his encouragement. From starting out trying to do in Peru what Paul did in Haiti, but then taking the other path to work on policy and politics and social movements, he had a fundamental impact on my career path. It was, to put it directly, to change from being a B-minus imitator of someone else, to being an authentic me. The greatest mentors hold up a mirror to you and say "be that person because I like that person." Howie took delight in talking to me—and he took delight in the person he saw and not the person he thought I should be. That's pretty profound. I really try to mentor with the spirit of Howard sitting on my shoulder, tell me what you love the most, not what you think you should be.

There were all sorts of particular details he helped us with, but more than anything else he helped us with tone: if I was getting too confrontational, or sometimes not tough enough. He was really a master of tone. It was the subtle management of human relationships that he was so good at, that there is a way of doing this, a way to bring about enormous, huge, powerful, change but doing it in a way that was thoughtful, civilized, a way of doing it so that you could remain friends, disagree but move forward. It was a preview of what adult life would look like. We thought we would speak truth to power. He gave me a completely different sense: speak truth to power but also manage relationships so that one day, you might find yourself in a position to change the world. And here I am.

"And here I am," said Jim Kim. In a recently published novel titled with these same words, *Here I Am*,[1] the author Jonathan Safran Foer has a character say it's "about who we are wholly there for, and how that, more than anything else, defines our identity." Howard Hiatt was wholly there for Kim, for Farmer, for Berwick. He was wholly there for his family. And he was wholly there for so many more across the generations. He was the model of a mentor.

Mark Rosenberg

What strikes me is how Howie has sustained his support for me and how much is has meant to me. I have known him for more than forty-five years. I first got to know Howard in my fourth year of medical school when I was living with my roommate, Harvey Fineberg, in an apartment on Mission Hill, in Roxbury. We decided that what we needed to round out our medical education was to invite a Harvard Medical School faculty member for dinner. We picked Howard Hiatt because he had been a leader in the medical community in opposing the Vietnam War, and advocating for the community—the one where we were living—in opposing a planned mega-expansion of the Peter Bent Brigham hospital, an incursion into the community that had been planned without any community input. Our apartment was always cold and neither of us really knew how to cook, but we didn't even know that we didn't know how to cook. Not only did Howard and his wonderful wife Doris come for dinner, but they even *ate* the chicken a l'orange that we had prepared. I was touched then, and now, that I know how much we didn't know about cooking and serving dinner to grown-ups, I am even more touched. He had a way of making me feel competent when I was way overextended.

I didn't see Howard much over the next two years as I was very absorbed in my medical internship and residency at Mass General, and I moved to Atlanta for two years where I tracked down enteric disease epidemics and smallpox at CDC. While in Atlanta I spent much more time on photography and decided that I would like to work on a documentary photography project that looked at what it was like to be sick, how it affected one's relationship with one's family, and what it was like to get medical care. I thought that having been a "sensitive" medical student, an intern and resident, and having covered the practice of a general practitioner on weekends for two years, I knew what it was like to be sick and I could show this to the world through the powerful medium of photography. Howard encouraged me, secured a grant to cover half of my salary, and created a position at the school of public health for me. I worked half-time on my photography documentary and taught courses in the Health Policy and Management program. When I had trouble getting permission from my old hospital, MGH, to take pictures of patients there—in 1976 there were very few images of sick people published—because they thought I would be airing medicine's dirty laundry in public, Howard intervened and arranged for me to be able to follow patients at the Beth Israel Hospital and the Brigham. When it came time to find a publisher, it was Howard who made the critical connection for me and then was so enthusiastic about my book.

When I had finished the book and had spent hundreds of hours photographing the six subjects of my book, their families and caretakers; talking to them about their experience; and just being with them—I realized then that when I had started the project I did not know what it was like to be sick or to be a patient. I knew what it was like to be a doctor, but I did not know what it was like to be a patient. I did not even know that I did not know. But Howard encouraged me to learn. He was able to make me feel that each new insight I acquired, each new lesson that a patient taught me, that these were remarkable discoveries and that I was discovering them for the first time. "Remarkable, Mark, what an amazing story and how wonderful for the patient that you were there to listen to them."

I left Boston, Beth Israel Hospital, and the Harvard School of Public Health and went back to CDC in 1983 at Bill Foege's request, to head up a new branch that was created to look at violence as a public health problem. Violence prevention was something new for public health and it did not prove to be an easy task. We were trying to apply science to the prevention of all sorts of violence—from child abuse and child sexual abuse to intimate partner violence, youth violence, suicide, and elder abuse. This was outside the mainstream of public health and my office showed it: my office was in the sub-sub-basement of building 3 in a room that had been converted from a men's room to an office. They had taken out the lavatory fixtures but all the plumbing still ran through it so that when anyone in the building flushed a toilet a river ran through it and you could not hear until it ran by. Throughout this time, Howard would reassure me saying "you are working on such an important problem, and what you find can do so much good for the whole country." So with reassurance from him and from Bill Foege, who by that time had stepped down as director of CDC, I pushed on. But as reassuring as he was, it didn't stop me from being fired twice for trying to push ahead in a bureaucracy that was not known for embracing change.

Howie was reassuring about problems at work and reassuring about problems at home. His highest praise was reserved not for finding a new way to look at suicide or the politics of gun violence, but for going to a soccer game practice with my kids, or going away for a weekend with my wife. Funny how people who are driven and hyper-focused on work have such good advice on how to balance family and work for others. Maybe we think we discovered it too late and want to help keep those we care about from making the same mistakes. At CDC we saw that injury was the leading cause of death for all Americans from one to forty-five and the two leading causes of injury death were guns and cars. Our government had been spending $200M a year on research to reduce road traffic deaths and this research had led to safer cars, safer roads, and safer drivers, saving more than 350,000 lives since the late 1960s. But although there were the same number of gun deaths as car crash deaths, the U.S. government was spending almost nothing at all on research to prevent gun deaths. So at CDC we started doing research to find ways to prevent gun deaths, gun homicides, gun suicides, and unintentional shootings. The NRA started paying attention to us, and criticized the work we were doing as "junk science." When the research we supported showed that having a gun in your home did not make you safer but actually increased by three to five times the risk that someone in your family would be shot and killed, the NRA was not happy. They didn't think this would help them sell more guns. They set out to shut us down, took away the funding we were using to support research on gun violence prevention, and did everything they could to make our work harder. Eventually they put pressure on a new director of CDC to get rid of me and I was fired. It was embarrassing and humiliating to be fired from a job into which I had poured my heart and soul.

But Howie was there with advice, comfort, and support. He never wavered, even at my most depressed times. When I left CDC, Bill Foege asked me to come work with him at a small global health nonprofit that he had started, the Task Force for Child Survival and Development. When I first got there in 1999, the task force was losing about $150,000 a year. The next year, Bill Foege left to go work with Bill Gates and start the Bill and Melinda Gates Foundation in Seattle, and he asked me to take over the Task Force. That year the Task Force had few assets other than our furniture. And all the furniture was used.

It was right about then, in 2000, that Howie suggested Jim and Paul call me to see if I could arrange for them to meet with Bill Foege and we set up that meeting at the Task Force. Jim and Paul went through their slides and Bill was impressed by them. That's when we started working together to put together a proposal for the Gates Foundation to fund their MDR-TB work in Peru. Howie came down for the first meeting of the partner organizations on the grant and when the meeting was over I drove my minivan with the four of us—Paul, Jim, Howie, and me—to celebrate at the best steak restaurant in Atlanta. I can still hear Paul yelling from the back to Howie in the front, "We did it, Howie. We fucking did it!" That was the beginning of our work on the Gates PARTNERS TB grant, a project that lasted seven years. Howie was our senior statesman, always willing to come to Lima for a special meeting whenever we needed someone dignified with impeccable credentials.

Howie served on the Task Force board of trustees for several years and came to Atlanta for our three-times-a-year meetings for several years. He was the only board member from out of town but he would come faithfully. Later he participated by phone. In those early years we struggled through some hard times. Howie never missed an opportunity to say something complimentary during the meetings. By 2015 the Task Force was doing much better. Our programs had grown to where we were receiving $3 billion a year in donations, mostly in the form of donated pharmaceuticals for our neglected tropical disease elimination programs. According to Forbes, the Task Force was the second largest charitable organization in the United States. That year Howie nominated us for the Hilton Humanitarian Prize, the largest humanitarian prize in the world. He nominated the Task Force and it won. What an incredible and humbling honor.

He always had a way of making me feel better about myself, and he affected me deeply and for a long time. As I have thought more about how this happened, I think that there are two parts to that. The first part is that we don't develop our strong beliefs based on rational arguments that we are presented with, but from relationships with people who mean a lot to us. This was best expressed by Daniel Kahneman, a man who won the Nobel Prize for his work on behavioral economics. In an interview with Krista Tippett he explained that

> The way that the mind works, very frequently, is that we start from a decision, or we start from a belief, and then the stories that explain it come to our mind. And the sequence that we have when we think about thinking, that arguments come first and conclusions come later, that sequence is often reversed. Conclusions come first, and rationalizations come later.

When I ask you about something that you believe in—whether you believe or don't believe in climate change or whether you believe in some political position or other—as soon as I raise the question why, you have answers. Reasons come to your mind. But the way that I would see this is that the reasons may have very little to do with the real causes of your beliefs. So the real cause of your belief in a political position, whether conservative or radical left, the real causes are rooted in your personal history. They're rooted in who are the people that you trusted and what they seemed to believe in, and it has very little to do with the reasons that come to your mind, why your position is correct and the position of the other side is nonsensical.[2]

The second part addresses the question of how can one single person have such a big effect on our life. The neuroscientist and psychiatrist Rachel Yehuda looked at what made the difference between people who were imprisoned during the Holocaust and survived and those who did not:

> "How are you?" has become a pleasantry that is devoid of all meaning. But just really kind of taking a second to inquire in a real way about how someone is doing. And even if they don't tell you, and even if they lie to you, it will probably have a beneficial effect. I mean, what I hear from trauma survivors—what I'm always struck with is how upsetting it is when other people don't help, or don't acknowledge, or respond very poorly to needs or distress. I'm very struck by that. And I'm very struck by how many Holocaust survivors got through, because it was one person that became the focus of their survival.[3]

If a single person could make the difference between life and death, it stands to reason that a single caring person in the form of a mentor can make a very large difference in someone's life.

I have a favorite song by the Kruger Brothers, a bluegrass group from North Carolina via Switzerland. I always think about Howie when I hear the words to this song. One day I was excited and called him up while the song was playing on the CD player in my car. I asked him to listen to something and held my phone near the speaker for him to hear:

> There's no reason to despair
> For there's always someone there
> Loves you more than you'll ever know
> Doesn't matter where you go
>
> When you find yourself alone
> In a world that's cold as stone
> In the darkness there's a light
> That will guide you through the night

> I think he thought I was a little crazy. I just said Howie,
> this is how I think about you.

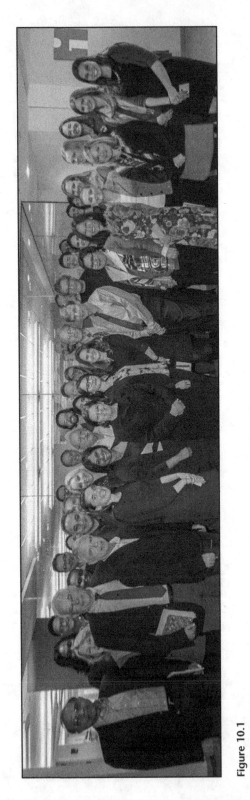

Figure 10.1

A meeting cosponsored by Global to Local and the Institute for Healthcare Improvement.

10 Bringing Global Health Home

A good mentor, Howard said, will have an opportunity to learn a tremendous amount from his or her mentees. And Howard was a good mentor. He put together several of the most important ideas he had learned at different stages of his career to develop a notion that he came to call Global Health at Home, a notion that came to be the focus of work in his ninth and tenth decades, when he remained very actively involved in mentoring. Even today, at ninety-two, he pursues continuous learning and thinks nothing of getting on a plane and crossing the country to visit two women physicians he is mentoring. In a single trip, he visited one of these physicians who was bringing preventive care and well-being to the Navajo nation in Gallup, New Mexico; then he went on to visit the other who was working in Los Angeles to incorporate the services of community health workers into preventive health programming. He went to learn from them, to see how they were doing, to encourage them, and to find out what he could do to help them.

These two young physicians were part of a movement that Howard pioneered and spread. Global Health at Home was built on a foundation that Howard constructed from his professional life across time and at different institutions. For example, at Beth Israel Hospital he transformed the department of medicine from a collection of physicians practicing the art of medicine as it had been passed on to them, into a science-based department founded on scientific research findings to which many in the department were actively contributing. From the school of public health came a focus on health systems and population health using quantitative methods to compare and analyze the effectiveness of different programs and approaches. He came away from the school of public health with the strong belief that the U.S. healthcare system was in need of improvement, and this improvement could be measured not only in terms of efficiency and cost but also in terms of equity. At Brigham and Women's Hospital, he saw that the more he worked with his wonderful mentees the more convinced he became that the value and techniques of global health held important potential applications in the United States. He came to believe strongly that we in the United States had a lot to learn from healthcare in other countries, particularly middle- and low-income countries where scarcity spurred innovation. And he believed that these lessons could be brought back to the United States, where they would improve health and healthcare. He also came to appreciate in this same way the idea of continuous improvement and continuous learning. This all came together to contribute to the notion of Global Health at Home, and Howard was central to this coming about. In 2015, Howard, Charlie Kenney, and I began a year-long exploration of how healthcare providers in the United States might learn from the lessons of global health. This chapter is the result of our discussions and draws heavily from the article "Global Health at Home: Harvesting Innovations from around the World to Improve American Medical Care," written by Howard, Charlie Kenney, and me, which first appeared in *Harvard Magazine*, November-December 2016.

We began by acknowledging that at its best, American medical care is a sublime blend of science and humanity, a system where doctors routinely transplant the human heart, replace defective joints, and excise tumors from the mid-brain. Every day in the United States, families are made whole again by some of the most complex surgical, medical, and pharmaceutical therapies ever devised, interventions from gifted physicians and researchers devoting their lives to alleviating human suffering. When political leaders declare, as many often do, that the United States has "the finest healthcare system in the world," it is this exalted aspect of American medicine to which they refer. So the notion that the United States might learn valuable lessons from care delivery in other nations—particularly poor countries—is instinctively counterintuitive to the pervasive belief that we have the finest healthcare on the planet.

Unfortunately, other aspects of American healthcare—lower quality and higher cost, as well as substantial health disparities—are considerably less uplifting. Such shortcomings leave the United States ranking at the bottom among the most advanced nations in comparisons of the quality and efficiency of care, even as the domestic cost of care (about $9,000 per capita), is double that of peer nations. The search is on for ways of delivering care in the United States that help improve the health and well-being of patients, effectively manage the health of populations, and are affordable. In this context, the assumption that U.S. healthcare is the "best" keeps us from learning valuable lessons about care delivery elsewhere. Our own experiences and research tell us that innovations in care are flowering throughout the world, and that these are ignored at great cost to Americans, many of whom are ill served by a health system that already accounts for one-fifth of the U.S. economy. Jim Yong Kim, while president of the World Bank, after having studied health systems around the globe, noted that it is well established that "situations of scarcity lead to innovation."

A good place to begin is by redefining what healthcare and public-health professionals in the United States now call "global health": improving conditions, particularly in poorer parts of the world, often by exporting expertise and resources from better-off areas like the United States and Europe.

At its best, global health implies an approach characterized by values, practices, and techniques that set it apart from the U.S. status quo. Beyond the care administered to the patients who come into a physician's office (or other parts of the formal health system, like hospitals), global health in this sense is premised on taking responsibility for *all* people in a given location—around the world, in the United States, and at all levels of income. Philosophically, global health is guided by the words of Paul Farmer: "The idea that some lives matter less is the root of all that is wrong with the world."

Equity is the soul of global health. In the United States, access to care—especially the very best care—is frequently correlated with ability to pay. Global health turns the focus from complex medical procedures and high-technology practice at the most advanced hospitals, per se, to the deployment of health and care resources throughout a large population of patients, recognizing that the lives of all people, whether wealthy or poor, possess equal intrinsic value.

This approach to health is patient centered. For decades, the doctor-patient relationship was at the center of the U.S. delivery system, but American healthcare has transitioned from patient centered to doctor centered and, finally, to payment centered. Global health marks a return to patient-centered care:

- In global health, caregivers take the time needed to understand and treat the patient and the context in which that patient lives. In that setting, a real relationship can develop between doctor and patient. In contrast, at a prestigious U.S. medical center, an ophthalmologist is rated based on whether she is able to complete sixty (!) patient visits per day, a schedule that doesn't allow the caregiver to know the patient, let alone the context.

- In global health, the patient is front and center. But U.S. caregivers too often find themselves required to spend valuable time responding to insurers' questions, time that could go to patient care.

- In global health, crucial determinants of well-being—poverty, unemployment, access to fresh food and clean water—are central to the caregiver's mission. But in U.S. medical practice, such factors typically fall outside clinicians' purview.

- In global health, local people possessing widely varying levels of skill and education—and often lacking even a rudimentary credential—play central roles in delivering care to individuals and promoting the community's health. But in U.S. medicine, credentials trump all and vast pools of potential talent go unused.

- More broadly, global-health practice shuns hierarchy in favor of inclusive teams—in sharp contrast to the determinedly hierarchical culture of U.S. hospitals and physician groups. Sprawling academic medical centers are suns around which many patients in the U.S. health system orbit. In global health, few large organizations get between caregivers and patients; care is delivered as close to the patient as possible—certainly in the community, and preferably in the home. The double meaning of global health at home helps define what we mean: applying global health ideas to care procedures in the United States—and sometimes, literally providing care in the patient's home.

In 1996, physicians from Brigham and Women's Hospital undertook to treat hundreds of patients in Lima, Peru, who had MDR-TB: highly infectious, often lethal and difficult to treat even under far more favorable conditions. MDR-TB was, in fact, so difficult to treat that the World Health Organization had pretty much given up on being able to stop this epidemic in poor countries. Paul Farmer and Jim Yong Kim were able to procure large quantities of medications for these patients, but they faced a difficult challenge: How could they make sure that all of the patients would take a combination of as many as seven medications—each with its own toxic side-effects—every day for as long as two years?

Their answer did not—indeed, could not—involve massive and expensive tertiary-care hospitals or highly credentialed academic physicians. The key, they found, was hiring local people to go to patients' homes daily to make sure they took their pills. These community health workers had little formal education and virtually no training, but they were a low-cost, extremely effective solution: women, recruited from the neighborhood, who knew the area and its culture well, and were able to gain the trust of patients. Through the community workers, Farmer and Kim and their clinical teammates learned about the reality inside patients' homes, enabling them to address needs for food, clean water, and transportation. In this case, an estimated 80 percent of patients were cured, a far higher rate than is typical even in the most advanced developed countries, and the cure came at a tiny fraction of the cost of treating MDR-TB cases in the United States.

"Global-health equity brings solutions to patients at their convenience," Farmer told us—particularly for chronic ailments. "We're not talking about home-based dialysis or interventional cardiology, but that's a small number of patients compared to people with chronic conditions. We need hospital-based care for those who are critically ill or injured, but for chronic conditions we want community-based care rather than clinic-based care."

This approach has also worked in the United States, particularly in disadvantaged settings. For example, consider how Heidi Behforouz, who trained at Brigham and Women's, took on AIDS. In 1997, during her first trip to central Haiti, she found that people with AIDS received care in their homes and were able to sustain a positive level of health and quality of life. But in Boston—the epicenter of the world's finest healthcare on the U.S. model— some AIDS patients received no care at all, while others relied upon periodic emergency-room visits when they became really ill. Behforouz and colleagues visited patients in several large, subsidized public-housing buildings near the hospital; there, she found many people suffering from a variety of highly treatable chronic conditions. "What struck me," she recalls, "was that people were dying in these buildings in this mecca of medical care, within walking distance of Harvard-affiliated hospitals. It didn't make any sense." What made sense, Behforouz thought, was to recruit and train people from the neighborhood to visit the sick, assess their situations, and deliver their medications. These recruits, she says, came to serve as "a bridge between the community and institutions which have become so professionalized and siloed that it's hard to establish therapeutic relationships." Those interventions improved health for thousands of people, reduced use of the Brigham and Women's emergency department, and thus reduced Medicaid costs for these patients by an estimated 35 percent. Better health, lower cost—and a model for the millions of U.S. patients who suffer common, chronic ailments (diabetes, heart failure, hypertension, and asthma) that can also be more effectively, and less expensively, addressed. Global health also came home to the Navajo Nation, 2,300 miles southwest of Boston, one of the reservations that in some ways, even more than the housing projects near the hospital, resemble less economically developed countries—places very far from the fortunate parts of the surrounding United States to which most of the payment-centered medical system caters.

Sonya Shin, a Brigham infectious-disease specialist, moved from Boston to New Mexico in 2009 to lead the Community Outreach & Patient Empowerment (COPE) partnership between the Navajo Nation, the Indian Health Service (a federal agency), Partners in Health, and the hospital. Like other Partners programs, she says, COPE employs "the same kind of philosophy of elevating the voice of the community members so they are part of the decision-making." Because resources and the number of health professionals were limited, she continues, "We relied upon grass-roots, community-based people. The strongest determinants of both disease and health outcomes exist in the community and have to be addressed in the community."

For example, Sarah Fatt, a fifty-four-year-old high-school graduate with a certificate as a nursing assistant, is now a community health worker engaged with COPE. She drives her pickup to her patients' homes in the Fort Defiance area of eastern Arizona, on the New Mexico border. When she arrives to examine eighty-four-year-old Julia M., the first part of the appointment resembles nothing so much as two old chums exchanging stories about family and friends: for the past ten years Sarah has helped Julia control her diabetes and hypertension. She measures Julia's blood-oxygen level and takes her temperature—movements choreographed through years of practice, now a natural accompaniment to their conversation. As Sarah reaches for a finger stick, Julia extends her hand.

Sarah observes that Julia is lucky to have family support from her son, daughter-in-law, and grandchildren, all of whom live nearby: "With diabetes, the family plays a huge role helping with food choices, taking walks, exercising, making sure she takes her meds." Through the years, she has educated

Julia and her family about diet, exercise, and medication. When Julia was confused about when to take certain medicines, Sarah sketched a drawing of the sun on one bottle to indicate that Julia should take it in the morning. On another, she drew a half sun for midday, and, on a third, she drew the moon. A year and a half ago, when Julia fell and broke a hip, the accident marked the first time since she began working with Sarah that she had been to an emergency room—and the only time she was admitted to the hospital. The contrast here is striking: Julia has managed her illness consistently and well, even as people throughout the United States with similar health problems—but whose conditions are not as well controlled—account for billions of dollars in avoidable spending on emergency visits and hospital stays.

Global to Local (G2L), a Seattle-area collaborative, demonstrates how these approaches can be applied beyond a single disease, to address community health more broadly. G2L defines its mission as bringing "strategies that have proven effective in developing countries to underserved communities in the United States," focusing on the diverse SeaTac and Tukwila communities, home to many immigrant families from Myanmar, Eritrea, Somalia, and nations throughout Latin America. G2L identified varied barriers to health: the unavailability of fresh fruits and vegetables, high unemployment, behavioral health challenges, and limited English-language skills. Most of the affected residents have limited formal education and find it difficult to navigate the complex healthcare delivery system. Rather than relying on traditional clinic- or hospital-based care, G2L focuses on using community health workers to understand the health needs in peoples' homes. It aims to link health to economic development (via public-private partnerships) and to integrate public health and primary care delivered in clinics. As an example, G2L focused on assisting diabetes patients by using smartphone-based applications: a simple but effective intervention to help them track diet, exercise, and blood sugars. The program also connected patients with student volunteers from the University of Washington who sent them text-message reminders to take their medications as well as notes of encouragement.

This low-cost program, requiring no physician or nurse time, yielded a significant improvement in enrolled patients' health. "The patients felt accountable to someone who cared about them," reports Adam Taylor, who directed the program. He says the students, who received some basic training, proved to be quite reliable and skilled in their dealings with patients.

The students also helped 7,000 people in the community complete the often-confusing work necessary to sign up for insurance under the Afford-able Care Act—one way to address broader public health issues.

Can a global-health approach also make a transformative difference among the tens of millions of well-educated, upper-income Americans, who commonly have access to insurance and higher-quality care?

Encouraging news on this front comes from the Pacific Business Group on Health (PGBH), a collaborative of large employers and government agencies based in California who use their insurance-purchasing clout to improve qual-ity and affordability. PBGH's "intensive outpatient care program" has focused on patients with multiple, complex chronic conditions who are frequent users of high-cost emergency-room visits and in-patient hospital stays. In the initial phase of the program, care coordinators visited 15,000 patients in twenty-three delivery systems in the western United States, seeking to establish trust-ing relationships with them. As this program continues, the idea is to have care coordinators visit patients in their homes and collaborate with the patients' primary-care physicians—providing medical care and addressing other needs (transportation, food) that have a direct bearing on health and quality of life. This integrated approach has resulted in significant improvements in both areas—and reduced emergency-room and in-patient stays.

PBGH's intensive outpatient care program has proven effective with large populations of well-educated, middle- and upper-income individuals. When tested among employees at Boeing suffering from a variety of medical con-ditions, hospital admissions decreased 28 percent. A similar approach with employees of the Pacific Gas and Electric Company and the California Public Employees' Retirement System has demonstrated that the intensive approach not only improves health and well-being but has also reduced claims costs by as much as 20 percent.

Whether in Haiti or in California, these successful approaches to improv-ing care all build upon caregivers who establish relationships with patients, go to their homes, and factor in broad determinants of health; all the approaches are, ultimately, patient centered. This care matrix can work in any setting, and can address the most pressing needs in the U.S. healthcare system: to improve the health and well-being of millions of Americans, at any income level, more effectively and efficiently. Global health improve-ments can work for the huge populations plagued by the kind of multiple, complex, chronic conditions that are epidemic in the United States.

What will be required to bring global health home to cure American healthcare? The obstacles are significant: tradition, culture, and regulations inhibit the kind of nimble innovation characteristic of the best global-health practices. Most doctors and caregivers aren't familiar with the strategies and services we describe.

But the timing is favorable for change. As generally rational economic actors, hospitals and physician groups do what they are paid to do. Under fee-for-service reimbursement, these actors have been paid for the volume of care they provide, rather than for its quality and outcome, producing well-documented overuse of clinical services. Global health seeks health as the outcome, not the volume of reimbursable services. Global health-driven innovations can also help the U.S. system absorb 20 million newly insured Americans. Because the Affordable Care Act prevents insurers from turning down people with pre-existing conditions, many of those recently enrolled are struggling with a variety of ailments. The global-health ethos of doing more with less, extending the care team to include community workers, and ministering to people in their homes as a way to improve their overall health, all align with current national needs.

Donald Berwick puts it this way: "We have to change the mentality of what excellence looks like. Excellence is not the gleaming new machine; it is someone who knows you and can help you access the resources and care you need from people you know." What he is talking about is global health; it is time to bring these improvements home to healthcare in the United States.

In March 2017, the Institute for Healthcare Improvement and Global to Local cohosted a conference at IHI in Cambridge to explore opportunities to bring global health home. It was driven by the shared belief that this concept has tremendous potential to improve health, improve healthcare, lower costs, and increase equity, as well as by the belief that it can benefit local, underserved communities. So the conference was designed to identify and bring together key thinkers and healthcare and public health leaders to move from believing in the concept of global health at home, to putting the values and principles into action. As Goethe said: Knowing is not enough; we must apply. Willing is not enough; we must do.

Among the broad questions that the group addressed were: How do we inventory the broad learnings of global health, share them widely, and actually apply them? How do we tailor approaches that have worked in one environment to a radically different one? How do we assemble partners who can collaborate to move from concept to action? Where does funding for this work come from? And how do we share our learnings and scale our successes?

We assembled an incredible group of participants for this meeting with experience spanning healthcare, global health, public health, public policy, funding, and place-based efforts that have started to test this concept of bringing global health home. The diversity of background and experience in this group, will, we hope, carry on and allow us to uncover the full potential of this approach and help pave the path forward. It will allow Howard to pass the baton, and, at ninety-two, change his status from Harvard professor to professor emeritus. And as he looked at this group that included some of the people he had mentored with such love, it looked like nothing could make him happier.

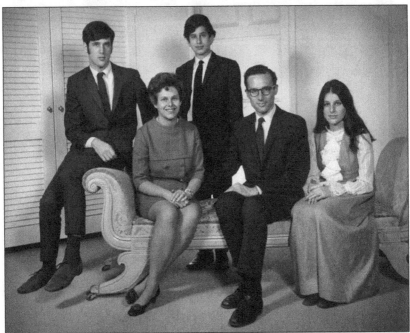

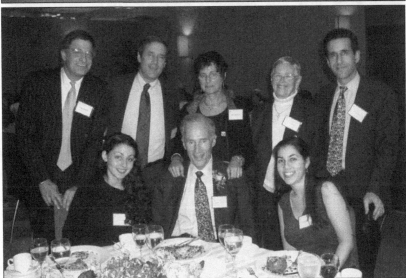

Figure 11.1

Top: Howard with his family on sabbatical in London (Harrods, 1969–1970). Left to right: Jon, Doris, Fred, Howard, Deborah. *Bottom:* Howard, Doris, and their children, Boston, October 2002. (Photograph by Harrod's, London.) Left to right: front row: Abby (Jon's younger daughter), Howard, Julie (Jon's older daughter); back row: Matt Epstein (Deborah's husband), Jon Hiatt, Deborah Epstein, Doris Hiatt, Fred Hiatt. (Photograph by Mark Rosenberg.)

11 Epilogue: A Fortunate Man

When we began this book, it told a story about a man who brought about change in three medical institutions and the very different experiences he had at each place. And it has, in fact, been largely a story about his life "at work," a life that has been very full and rewarding. But Howard's professional life has been only one thread in an even fuller life, a life in which work and family intertwined. They were not totally parallel and they were not divergent. It was the thread of his family life that made it possible for his work thread to engage him, hold him, and support him without breaking, becoming part of a thicker, stronger thread that not only endured but grew stronger. For this Howard sees himself as a very fortunate man.

I trust that my great good fortune with respect to teachers, colleagues and students is apparent. But I have had even greater good fortune in my family—my wife, Doris; our three children: Jon, Deborah and Fred, and their spouses, whom both Doris and I considered our equally loved children; their children, our grandchildren: Julie, Abby and Michael Hiatt, Eric and Andrea Epstein; Alexandra, Joe and Nate Hiatt. But at the heart of all my great good fortune is Doris. She and I met when she was a Wellesley senior and I was a third-year Harvard medical student. Early on, I was not at all certain that I was prepared to make a permanent commitment at that stage of my life and medical career. That uncertainty was sensed by Doris's mother, Gertrude Bieringer, a remarkable and perceptive woman of whom I was to become a great and warm admirer. On the evening that we decided to marry, Doris phoned her parents to tell them the news. Gertrude asked to speak to me, and Doris passed the phone over. With steel in her voice, Gertrude asked, "Howie, are you sure?"

About few things in my life have I ever been more sure. It would be difficult to project what my life would have been like without Doris. She was, without question, the most supportive person I ever knew. She was extraordinarily insightful—the decisions that I made with respect to my own career were far sounder than they would have been had they not been discussed at length with her. She provided a constant model, close at hand, of deep sympathy with and commitment to (not necessarily the same thing) the problems of people less fortunate than she. One example that was especially meaningful to me was her choice of a 75th birthday present. Shortly before that birthday, Doris had a total remission following her first bout of lymphoma. Our daughter, Deborah, had a party to celebrate the birthday and the remission.

I thought that an appropriate birthday present would be a new car to replace her fifteen-year-old Honda. Doris declined. "My car works perfectly well," she said. So, I gave a sum equivalent to the cost of a new car to Horizons for Homeless Children, the wonderful organization whose board Deborah's husband, Matt, chaired for several years. The Horizons director gave me twenty drawings of a car to give to Doris, each drawn by one of the homeless children. Doris was delighted. She said it was "the second-best birthday present I have ever received." (I knew well that the first was the birth of Fred, the youngest of our three children, on her 31st birthday.)

While his family was incredibly important to him, Howard never aspired to achieve the perfect work-life balance. When he was working at Beth Israel Hospital and at the Harvard School of Public Health, this subject was not quite as top-of-mind as it is today. But Doris held a special place:

Beyond all else, Doris put aside her own wishes and aspirations to support and promote me. I wince when I think of the number of times that she gave up something she wanted to do because she felt it might interfere with my plans. In the days when we had but one car, she would often come pick me up at the end of the day to have dinner with our children. I thought little of keeping her waiting outside my office for fifteen or twenty minutes or, I hate to say it, even longer. When she raised a question about a particularly lengthy delay, I had only to mention a patient suddenly in need of my attention or a medical student who had shown up with a problem that couldn't wait and she would either accept this without question or, rarely, shake her head very slightly and then go on to something else.

It was almost routine for me to return to my lab or to my office after dinner while she cleaned up and put the children to bed. When I watch my sons and daughter with their spouses and realize how evenly their household chores are divided, I am embarrassed at what I—and Doris—accepted as normal. It is true, of course, that the culture has changed considerably, but it seems to me now that my behavior was extreme in its assumption that I was the important partner in the marriage.

When she felt that our children no longer needed her close supervision, Doris and a friend, Celeste Klein, a bibliophile like Doris, decided that the availability of good paperback books was not getting sufficient attention from high school librarians. They launched KLIATT, a quarterly review of newly published paperbacks for the Young Adult audience. With the help of college student reviewers,

KLIATT, distributed throughout the country, expanded the interest in the newly available (and less expensive) paperback books at school libraries often suffering the effects of funding cutbacks.

As the many books sent to KLIATT by hopeful publishers piled up, Doris and Celeste first handed them out to anybody who was interested and then discovered David Mazor, a man in Amherst, MA, who would deliver them in quantities to impoverished high school libraries, mostly in western Massachusetts. He began a program enlisting Amherst students to read with students at these high schools. Called Reader to Reader, it provided copies of a book to a college student and a high school student and they would "read" the book together, using email to discuss it. After Doris's death, I decided that no memorial would be more appropriate than to make it possible for the program to continue and to expand. Thus, the Doris Hiatt Mentoring Program has now spread beyond Massachusetts to schools in Alabama and on the Navajo Reservation in New Mexico. David has reported that many students have shown increases in their enjoyment of reading, and a number of high schools have reported improvement in reading scores.

Howard takes great pride in how much he has learned from those he has mentored. But he takes his greatest pleasure in recognizing how much he has learned and how much his life has been enriched by his children and their families—every day.

Our children enriched our lives in many, many ways, demonstrating the kind of strong values and commitments that have made me proud to be their father. Jon, who has always cared passionately about standing up for the rights of those who are too easily exploited, trained in labor law and was for many years director of the legal department and subsequently the number two at the AFL-CIO. Over one stretch of time, while fulfilling his administrative duties in Washington, he would take night flights to and from Los Angeles to encourage and monitor the organization of car washers into a union. Jon married Barbara Shepp, his college classmate, a social worker who worked with women victims of domestic abuse. Deborah worked after law school with the families of coal miners in Kentucky, but after a few years had to give up the law for medical reasons. She has become a serious painter. She married Matt Epstein, who combines work with a large Boston law firm with extensive community service, especially with Horizons for Homeless Children, where he served as chair of the board for a number of years, and as a leading board member of Beth Israel Deaconess Hospital.

Fred as a Harvard student wrote for the Crimson and rose to be Associate Managing Editor. He married Margaret ("Pooh") Shapiro—who was Managing Editor. Fred and Pooh have spent their lives in journalism, mostly at the *Washington Post*, for which they have reported both domestically and abroad (Japan, then Russia). David Broder, one of the paper's most respected political reporters, once told me that nobody had done more for the *Post* than Fred, because when he was sent to Tokyo as Bureau Chief, he said he would not do it unless Pooh were made Co-Chief. "She is so much better as a manager than I am," he told his bosses. This was, Broder told me, an important change for the *Post*. Fred is now the Editorial Page Editor at the paper, and Pooh, after time off to focus fully on raising their three children, edits the health and science sections.

I can say with total candor that I don't resent in the least that Joe, an MD-PhD student at UCSF Medical School, seems to be the only one of this marvelous group who has chosen to follow their grandfather's career. And my good fortune has continued with Penny Janeway, who has been my partner since Doris's death, and the arrival of Caroline Calliope Hiatt Hanlon, Abby's daughter, my first great-grandchild.

Words about the good fortune my family has provided would be incomplete without mention of my closest friend, my brother, Arnold Hiatt. From a childhood so contentious that our father once brought home a pair of boxing gloves with instructions to us to "take it downstairs to the basement," Arnie has become the friend whom I most admire and on whom I most depend. Paul Farmer once referred to him as "Howard's accompagnateur," the Partners in Health word for the community health worker who travels with a patient through his or her disease and treatment. For me, Arnie has been that, and more.

It is not clear that anyone achieves the perfect work-family balance. Although there are many people who claim to have done this and are eager to share the secrets of their success with us. They would have us believe that we walk through life with a bucket in each hand; we just have to put the same amount of weight in each bucket to achieve a perfect balance, and, once we have achieved this balance, just walk steadily forward without spilling anything. But this is probably the wrong image. This balancing act is more like trying to balance oneself while walking a tightrope or doing exercises while balancing on a rubber hemisphere—it is inherently unstable and requires attention on a daily basis.

But Howard has had an opportunity to become increasingly engaged with his growing family—which now includes a great-granddaughter—over the last decade or two, certainly between the ages of seventy and ninety-two, an opportunity that most people never get, and a chance to achieve a balance over time, a chance that most people also don't get. And for this he considers himself a very, very fortunate man indeed.

12 A Life Remembered

I had the good fortune to be able to look at these pictures with Howard when he was ninety-two. It was a chance to ask him what they brought to mind and what he remembered, and to think about what were the things he felt meant the most. Daniel Kahneman, a social psychologist who won the Nobel Prize in economics for his work on behavioral economics, spoke with Krista Tippett about the difference between life as we experience it and life as we remember it.

Daniel Kahneman: Well-being is something that you experience every second of your life: You are more or less happy. You are in a better or worse mood. And you can recall that continuously, and that's the well-being of the experiencing self. But then, there is another way of measuring well-being, which is to stop people and to ask them to think about their life and to say whether their life is good or bad. It's completely different. That's the well-being of the remembering self; it's an act of memory and construction. And the two are quite different.

Krista Tippett: Does one of these, the experiencing self or the remembering self, always trump the other, or is that a different dynamic in any given life?

Daniel: No, that's the interesting part, I think. When I started out in this line of research, I was a strong believer that the reality of life is what the experiencing self is. I mean it's what happens as you live. And I thought that's vastly more important than what people think about their life, which, after all, is a construction. And I went about defending the experienced well-being as the more important one. And eventually, I had to change my mind.

And I had to change my mind and conclude that there is no way you can ignore remembering self or life evaluation, because what people want is not the well-being of their experiencing self. What people want is more closely associated with the remembering self. They want to have good memories. They want to have good opinions of themselves. They want to have a good story about their life.[1]

The work that was done on most of the chapters for this book was an attempt to accurately portray the way that Howard experienced his life. But talking about these photographs was a chance to find out much more about how Howard remembered his life and to hear the story that he had about his life when he was ninety-two.

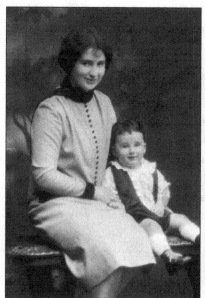 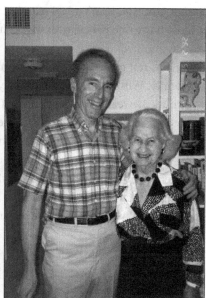

Howard with his mother, and Howard and Dorothy many years later.

Howard Hiatt: How beautiful a woman my mother was and what a difficult early life she had. She lived with a very difficult man, my father. When this picture was taken she was probably not yet twenty years old. She had left high school to work to help support her family. It was just extraordinary that a person with the disadvantages that she had really did what she did. The respect and affection that people showed for her—whether it was the person in the coffee shop or the janitor—she was just so caring.

She had to manage a household—I was the oldest of three children and my father was not very helpful in the home and he was not very gentle in his relations with my mother—so I really had a sense of the difficulties that surrounded her. When I was a good deal older, when I was a medical student, I became quite angry at my father when he had been very critical of her. I told him I didn't find that acceptable behavior. He was a difficult man and she bore the brunt of that difficulty.

His life had not been an easy one. He left a home in Eastern Europe with eight siblings and came alone before his fifteenth birthday to this country. His parents and four of his siblings and their families were murdered in the village where they lived in Lithuania not by the Nazis but by the non-Jews in that area. He wasn't a bad man but had a difficult life and wasn't able to deal with the one person over whom he early on had complete control: that was my mother.

He was not a very generous person in his dealings with persons outside the family. Within it he was extremely helpful and kind.

I think he really was respectful of the fact that at school I was almost always ahead of the class and that meant a good deal to him. He thought that was important. Was he kind, generous and supportive of me? I don't know how to answer that question, but I do know that one of the kindest, most generous people whom I know, whose kindness and generosity are kept secret some of the time, is my brother and my father's behavior toward him was not kind or generous. How to put all that together is very difficult to think about.

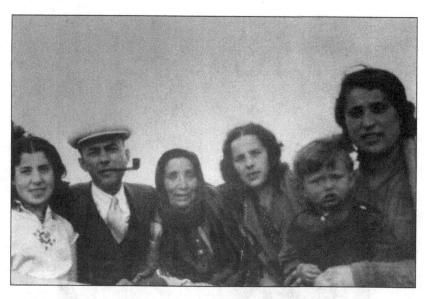

Howard's father with his mother, three sisters, and nephew.

Howard: My father went "home" once, and that was when I was about five or six years old. He went to Obilai or Obel. He was from a family of four sisters and five brothers. He brought all but one of his brothers here to the U.S. None of the sisters wanted to come so he went home to see his mother and sisters. His sister Goldie was in a concentration camp; her child and her husband were murdered but she survived. When the war was over she went home to Lithuania to find out what happened to her family. She found that all of them—except one who went to a concentration camp—had been murdered by the non-Jews living there. Her husband and child were murdered by the Nazis.

I was in medical school when I learned that the people my father had gone to visit had been murdered. It was a profound shock to have that news. My parents acknowledged the existence of a virulent anti-Semitism in Europe and elsewhere, including the U.S., so, this was not something unexpected from their point of view. I would be hard put to say that any of this with respect to my family had a profound effect on either my outlook or activities. Who knows, Greta Bibring might feel differently about that. [Greta Bibring was a psychoanalyst who became the first woman full professor åt Beth Israel Hospital and Harvard Medical School.]

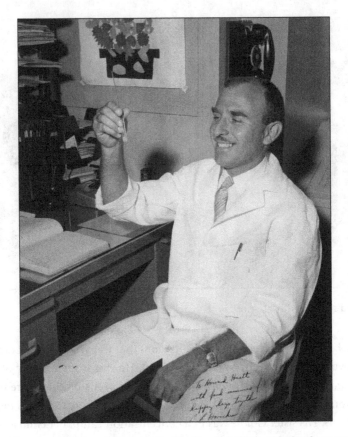

Bernie Horecker. The inscription reads: "To Howard Hiatt with fond memories of happy days together. B.L. Horecker."

Howard: I have told you more than once how crucial a person he was in terms of my own development and that picture evokes that sense. Absent Bernie my career would have been very, very different and not nearly with the gratification that it has had, or with some of the difficulties. Because absent the background in science I would probably never have been given the chairmanship of medicine at Beth Israel and absent that I would not have had the chance to build what I did there. I would not then have had the offer of the School of Public Health or any of the other deanships that I was not prepared to take.

I got to Bernie Horecker's lab quite by chance. When I arrived at the NIH the clinical laboratories in the clinical center weren't quite completed. An acquaintance urged me to meet Bernie Horecker. He greeted me warmly and I suggested a friend thought he might have room for me in the laboratory. He said he had. I learned how science was done by a person of great skill and great generosity. Later, when I was offered a position in Boston by Hermann Blumgart, and accepted the offer, I told Bernie what I wanted to do. He said there is no reason we can't stay in close touch. And we did. After a couple of years at Beth Israel, he said "you are now running the cancer program at Beth Israel and if you want to go deeper the new area of molecular biology is what you need to learn about. I have just come back from the Institute Pasteur in Paris and if you are interested I can make arrangements for Jacques Monod to take you for a year." Throughout his life we stayed in close touch. He took great pleasure in seeing my papers. He took great pleasure in what you were able to do and succeed at. It was that sort of thing that led me to understand what mentoring really means. when people ask me how I explain the fact that there were a number of people that I helped, I have told the Horecker story as how I learned what mentoring means and how it could be carried out.

Mark Rosenberg: What do you see in Bernie Horecker's picture?

Howard: I see a man of great curiosity, of persistence, of kindness and who made significant contributions scientifically and in terms of the younger people with whom he had relationships. So this was a model for me, something that not too many people have an opportunity to experience. How was he different from my father? There was really no comparison. When you understand that my father came penniless to this country and had the experience he did, you understand to at least some extent what lay behind his behavior.

Mark: A neuroscientist and psychiatrist, Dr. Rachel Yehuda found that for holocaust survivors what made the biggest difference—between survival and death—was to have one person who cared about them and was kind. It strikes me that this applies to mentoring where the mentor is the person who cares and is kind. Life is hard for everyone, even if it is not a question of life and death.

Howard: I share that sense. With Bernie it was really profound. That notion that one person can make a difference, it certainly had that effect on me. Not long ago, when the chairman of medicine at UCSF introduced me as the person who has mentored more people than anyone else he knew—that was a great surprise because I don't look at myself as someone who has had a profound effect on others but as someone who has been very fortunate to have had contact and access to people like Don and yourself.

People have from time to time, expressed awareness of my having mentored some younger people and when I am asked to go beyond that, my answer is almost always that the mentor that I had was so important in my life that I couldn't not be moved by that in the relationships with the younger people with whom it has been my privilege to have relationships.

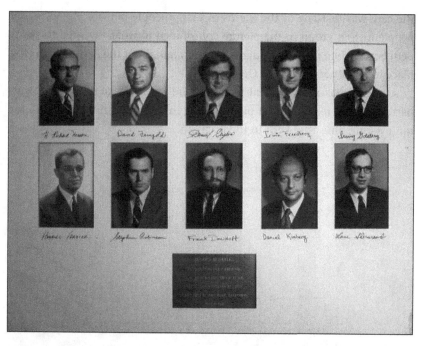

Hiatt's Hoplites. *Hoplites* is a Greek term meaning "heavily armed foot soldiers." This composite photograph of all of Howard's division directors whom he recruited to the department of medicine at Beth Israel Hospital was presented to Howard upon his leaving Beth Israel Hospital in 1972 to assume the deanship at the Harvard School of Public Health. The inscription reads: Hiatt's Hoplites/Recollecting old campaigns/ and anticipating those to be,/although untutored in pride,/still feel it, and more, affection./June 12, 1972

Howard: I love that picture. There are periods in my life that I look back on with enormous pleasure. I don't have to tell you that the period at SPH is not in that category. The period with Bernie Horecker is surely in that category. My time with the group of colleagues whom I recruited to the Beth Israel Hospital is in that category. A marvelous group of people. They were enthralled in caring for patients and doing extremely interesting research but also being gifted doctors. They were known as a group of caring, very skillful doctors who were leaders in their fields and leaders in their attitudes toward their patients and their students. It's a period of my life that I look back on as being quite marvelous.

When I started, Beth Israel Hospital was the local Jewish Hospital and the community knew it. Some of the people at Harvard Medical School felt that the care was first-rate at the hands of many people but not all. So, many people in that group in the picture contributed to what I wanted to see at Beth Israel, when medical students began to talk about the Beth Israel as the place to go rather than Mass General.

At the school of public health this picture was a crucial thing to look at, particularly there. Later, that picture hung in my office in the Brigham for quite a long time after I got to the Brigham.

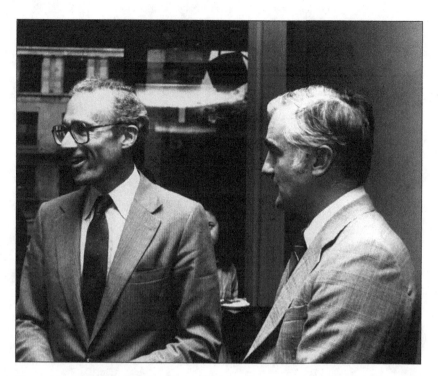

Howard Hiatt and Derek Bok

I should tell you that my reaction to Derek and to this offer he made to me, and my having accepted that offer, really was not wholly dependent on what I am about to say but certainly wouldn't have taken place absent that. And that is that Derek cared. He wanted a school of public health to be what it wasn't when he started, and he was quite sympathetic when he asked me to take that position. I am not in any way indicating that what I am talking about as caring is limited to physicians nor is it necessarily an attribute of all physicians. But I think Derek Bok saw the school of public health as one place where his leadership of the university could be expressed in a way that reflecting his caring. This was not restricted to the school, but the program, teachings and research of the school could reflect this to a greater extent than any of the other schools for which he was responsible. And he discovered very soon that that wasn't the way the school was being used or wasn't so regarded by people.

Mark: Are you saying he cared about the people who could benefit from the school? Are you saying he shared, with you, a similar compassion?

Howard: I am, I do.

Mark: Do you think this panned out?

Howard: By and large I do.

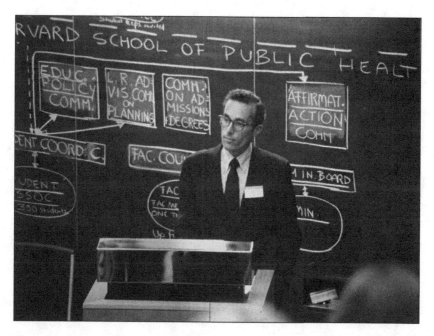

Howard in front of a blackboard diagram.

Howard: I look younger than I feel today. It looks as though I am looking for ideas and the last one that was offered doesn't strike me as the one I was after. And why am I not in New Haven as we are speaking now? I look at myself, presumably as the dean, talking with faculty about what we are really confronting. We are dealing with a series of complex problems, and we are going to have to spend more time thinking about the school as a whole rather than as departments. We met with each department head for a full day during that summer. The question was how to address the needs of the field and try to build a faculty and a school here that would lead or at least take an important role in meeting that need. At the end of that summer I remember saying to Doris how did I manage to get myself into this? If I had had that knowledge when I first got Derek's offer I never would have done it. I was now stuck, I had no choice. I had accepted Derek's offer, turned down Yale's offer.

I do think it was a mistake for having taken the position. For these reasons. I gave up an opportunity to develop the needs of a medical school, and a great one under the leadership of a great president at Yale. Second, it was a school that was in great need of rehabilitation or building and there was no doubt then about what it needed. But was that how I wanted to spend the next five years—or what I thought I was committed to? I had no choice but to move forward in that situation. And how to go about it pretty much alone. I found, at least at that time, nobody at the school who was going to assist in the building process. Lots of people who felt that there wasn't any building that was necessary. They had succeeded in getting rid of my predecessor at the school and he was one of them. All of that was a pretty unhappy time. In retrospect after a short time there was a growing group of people I had recruited and who made a great difference. But at that time, I had no idea of how I could do that. So, it was a grim time.

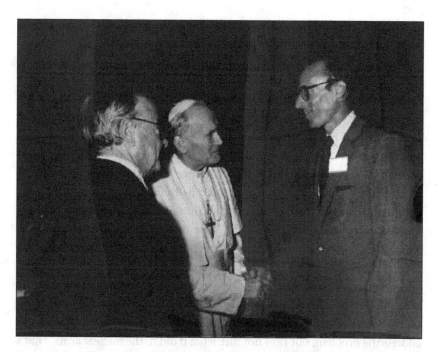

Carlos Chagas Filho, Howard, and Pope John Paul II, December 1981. "President Reagan took time Tuesday to meet a Vatican-sponsored delegation headed by Dr. Howard H. Hiatt, dean of the School of Public Health, that urged an increased effort to abolish nuclear weapons. The meeting was the first of several that will take place between emissaries of Pope John Paul II and leaders of four of the five recognized nuclear powers. Hiatt and three other experts told the president that casualties from a single megaton explosion in Washington, D.C., would overwhelm the area's medical facilities, a suggestion Reagan reportedly did not dispute. Hiatt said that Reagan acknowledged during the twenty-minute meeting that a nuclear exchange would 'end civilization as we know it' and that it is impossible to 'reconcile this with thoughts that one can win or survive a nuclear war.'" From the *Harvard Crimson*, December 18, 1981.

Howard: This picture was taken at a time when there was great worry about the possibility of a nuclear war. And not nearly as much danger then as now. Because both physicians and other scientists in several countries had focused on the issue of nuclear war, Chagas, who was head of the Pontifical Academy of Sciences, suggested that he bring people together from what were then the four nuclear powers—US, France, Britain and the Soviet Union. Because I had been pretty active as a physician in that effort and had some conversations with Dr. Chagas, who was Brazilian, I was invited, along with three other Americans—two Nobel laureates, David Baltimore, Marshall Nirenberg, and Viki Weisskopf, a professor at MIT.

There were similar numbers of prominent people from the other countries, leading figures in their fields. We were asked to prepare a paper that the pope could use as a kind of encyclical that he could send to the heads of the four states. After the first day we agreed that the paper should focus on the medical implications of nuclear war. Because I was a physician who had focused on that subject I was asked to do most to the writing. The pope than asked the leader of each country to meet with the people he had met with at the Vatican. So a few weeks later, Baltimore, Weisskopf, Nirenberg, and I met with Reagan. The meeting with Reagan was really quite distressing because it was clear that he had little interest in meeting with us but couldn't turn down this request from the pope. Since the message from the pope was largely focused on the medical consequences of nuclear war, my colleagues asked me to speak with Reagan. This was a front-page story in the *NYT* and the *Washington Post* and elsewhere. What happened was more than a little sobering. The pope was clearly eager to do what he could to address the problem, but I am not sure what it did to the nuclear arms. That's more important today as I think about how little care or caring or concern that our present leader has. We think about ourselves and our children and their children—because it is really about them—and see how relatively little attention this issue is getting in the White House, it is frightening. It is really just so dangerous. Looking back at the picture I see how much attention a person like the pope, with as much international power—power not in any sense other than his influence over people—how much attention that issue received from this powerful man. And how fortunate I was to be able to offer my impressions to him and perhaps to strengthen whatever feelings he had about the problem.

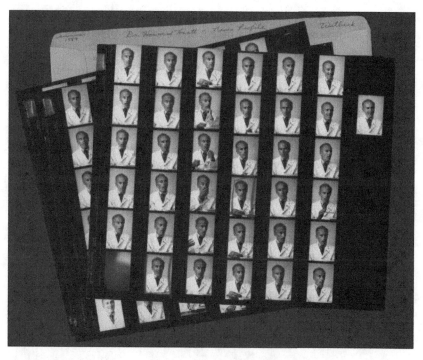

Contact sheet of Howard Hiatt in Brigham and Women's Hospital white coat. (Photo by David Whitbeck)

Howard: When I took the bureaucratic position as a dean I lost the opportunity to interact on a one-on-one basis with people in need of medical care or in need of compassion. Now you can say that I really focused in a bureaucratic sense on people with such needs when I went to the school of public health. But as you know that is not the same. When you are in the presence of a person in need of medical care and you are in a position to provide that medical care, an element of gratification accompanies the fact that you are able to be responsive. At the school of public health, just to simplify, you are dealing with that individual but in large numbers. You are dealing with a population with those needs, and the outcome of what you do can often offer a similar kind of gratification. But it lacks something important. So when I got back to the Brigham it was a chance to rehabilitate myself in medicine. Wearing a white coat had more than symbolic value because I worked in one of the primary care clinics and while I wasn't able to do all that I wanted to do, I had a few patients and was consulted about others so I was able to become a physician again. I had a chance to find out again how a hospital worked, some of its problems, some of its opportunities.

We had planned to look at the problems of medical injury and what could be done to both prevent the problems and prevent the consequences of the problems. That was my first undertaking after I left the school of public health. So I was at the Brigham and together with Lucien Leape and Frank Weiler, a professor of law, we carried out the medical practice study, which Don [Berwick] says was the basis for what he did at the IOM on medical errors. Lee Goldman and I talked about introducing the fellows in cardiology to concepts in quantitative analysis and what it might make possible in medical education. That program now takes 170 students a year who are physicians at the medical school and the school of public health.

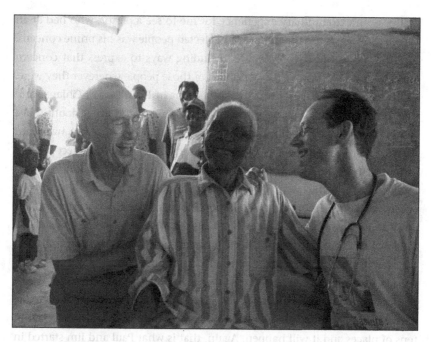

Howard and Paul Farmer laughing with a 104-year-old man in Haiti, 2004. In rural Haiti, this man walked six miles to see his doctor, Dr. Paul Farmer. He said he was 104 years old, and he really was. At first he told us that he had come because he had pain in his legs, but after "Doctor Paul" examined him and found nothing wrong with his legs, he admitted that he had walked all that way to see his doctor because just seeing Doctor Paul made him feel better. (Photo by Mark Rosenberg)

Howard: This man came to see Paul at a clinic near Cange in Haiti. He told me that his grandchildren had grandchildren. It really must have been a struggle to survive all that time in the conditions to which he was exposed. Paul's activities in Cange were as remarkable in many ways as Paul himself is. He was not only the doctor, but he was the person who discovered the area as a potential site initially for a school and subsequently for the hospital. He saw to it that trees were planted all around and this had been not years but decades before. In addition, he helped in the dissemination of that pattern of the hospital in Cange

It represents an overview of the remarkable achievements of a unique man. I don't use that word very often because it is so often misused. But when it is applied to Paul it is not misused at all. There is no one like him or even close to him.

It was an extraordinary experience for me to see a person who had at an early age decided that the welfare of neglected people was his prime concern. And that he would devote his life to finding ways to express that concern and find ways to improve the condition of those people wherever they were. In his instance, it was not just in Haiti, it was in Peru, and in Chiapas and subsequently in many places in Africa. Without Paul and Jim, I doubt that I would have gone in the direction of global health. They not only awakened me to what I was conscious of, but in great detail. Not only the abject poverty of hundreds of millions of people, but that there are ways to address those problems and in that way, bring benefit to millions of people. And further, to recruit younger people to walk in their footsteps. That's what Paul and Jim and I must say, Victor Dzau, in initiating the residency, did. The residency in global health has led to not just a group of people who are committed to the well-being of those people but who are committed to creating the circumstances where the well-being of those people is an objective and where the other doctors can be recruited to join in that effort. I know that there are global health residents all over the world now, not literally of course, but in tens of places and it will happen. Again, that is what Paul and Jim started in Haiti.

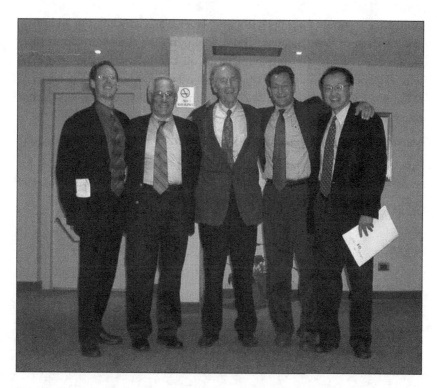

Four brothers. Howard came to speak at a meeting in Lima, Peru, in 2001 where Paul Farmer, Don Berwick, Mark Rosenberg, and Jim Kim were working together on a project to show that multi-drug-resistant tuberculosis (MDR-TB) could be treated effectively and at a low-enough cost to make treatment feasible for poor people in resource-poor settings. (Photo by Mark Rosenberg)

Howard: Compassion, improving the plight of the poor. They did share compassion, they do share that. Certainly my reaction to any suggestion that this was a goal for any one of them when he and they mentioned goals—and that happened with some frequency—my reaction immediately, of course, was one of great enthusiasm. But, no surprise, because anyone who really knew Paul or Jim or Don or Mark would have known at once well what their attitude was and remained about disenfranchised people, people in need of whatever.

Mark: Compassion would also describe you, would it not?

Howard: I didn't go to Hopkins as dean because I couldn't get the senior faculty to agree that the welfare of people in their neighborhood was a concern and should have been not only labeled as a concern, but addressed as a concern of their medical school. I couldn't get the chairman of their trustees, Gus Long, the president of an oil company, to agree that Harlem was not only an appropriate and essential neighbor, but a concern of Columbia's medical school. I don't have any difficulty acknowledging that that has been on my agenda, as it has been on yours.

Mark: Do you think that compassion has been a value that has guided you?

Howard: It certainly has been among what I look for and have looked for in my career, in the situations in which I have found myself, what I looked for in my colleagues, what I used to guide myself.

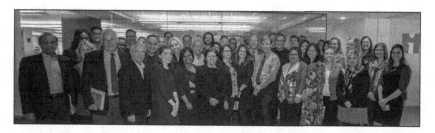

Picture of Global Health at Home. Sixty people came together at a meeting cosponsored by Global2Local, a nonprofit in Seattle and the Institute for Healthcare
Improvement in Cambridge, Massachusetts, to discuss and plan for moving forward with Howard Hiatt's vision of bringing global health home. There were few
things that made Howard happier than to plant ideas with energetic young people
who were committed to improving health and healthcare for all. (Photo by Rebecca
Goldberg)

Howard: It is a big picture of a big group. You look at this picture and you
see at least some of the marvelous people that it's been my good fortune
to know and to work with and how magical they are in attracting people.
Because most of the individuals in that picture are there because of them:
Don, Maureen, Sonya, Mark and others also. That's been part of my good
fortune.

Mark: To me this represents you passing the idea of Global Health at Home
on to new generations.

Howard: You are extremely generous in your reading that picture that way,
and wouldn't I be an ingrate if I rejected out of hand your interpretation.
There's Mark and the people he attracted. It's pretty wonderful. There are
a couple of graduates of the Global Health Residency there so when I look
at that picture and I recognize Don's face and Sonya's face, there are others
that I recognize, I just feel so fortunate.

I have on my desk a letter that arrived the day before yesterday from
Sonya Shin that began "I want to express my deepest appreciation and
gratitude for everything you are doing for COPE. Your support for restor-
ative justice for Native Americans has been a beacon of hope for COPE."
How rewarding it is to have a note like that from someone like Sonia. It is
true I am lucky, as I keep telling you, and that luck is expressed and mani-
fest in a range of ways, none perhaps more meaningful that the relationship with the person I am talking with right now.

Mark: I wanted to help you see your life as an arc that led to the position you find yourself in now, where you see the arc of your life as that of a very fortunate man.

Howard: My relationship with Mark Rosenberg says so much and I wish that this weren't so expensive in time to him. But it has been that and I am grateful for it.

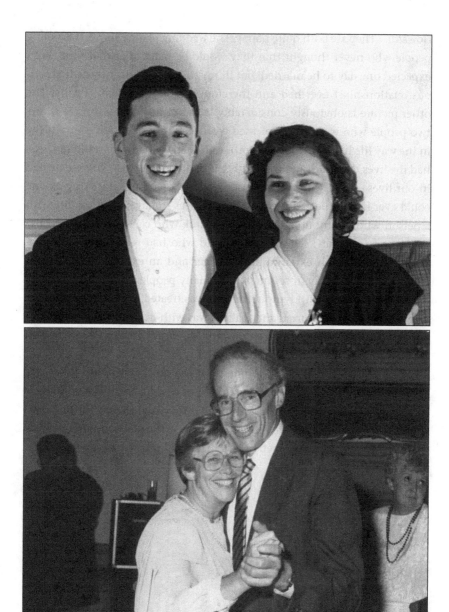

Howard and Doris on the day before their wedding, and Howard and Doris dancing fifty-three years later.

Howard: They are both quite happy. The wedding picture shows two young people who never thought that they would be married at that time. Both expected one day to be married, but in my instance Doris was the first serious relationship I ever had and therefore the only one until Penny. The other picture is obviously considerably later in our marriage and it shows two people who were rather pleased with each other and felt pretty lucky in the way life had treated them both. And then we had three children who had the lives they had, and they had children. And the way we were treated in our lives—all of this was about as rewarding, happy, gratifying as one could ever have expected. How fortunate I was to have spent my life with a person whose attributes were so wonderful, who cared so deeply, whose values were all that I felt and more. And who had really been an extraordinary partner, an extraordinary mother and an extraordinary human being who really brought so much to so many people.

She was stricken with lymphoma that was treated, we thought, successfully initially but it recurred and really it was with her and me for—I didn't remember exactly how long—not months but more. It was a loss to me and to our children and to their children.

As I look back I feel that the time went too quickly between those two pictures. In terms of our children neither of us could have imagined that we would have the enormous good fortune that they, and their 3 partners, and their children would have brought us. Those were the most important events that characterized our life together and that really superseded anything else.

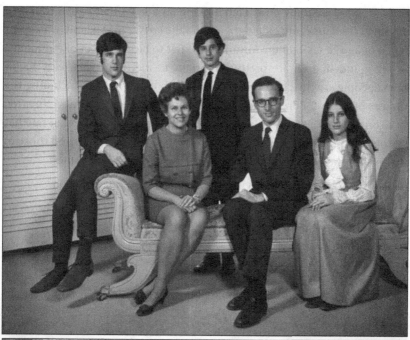

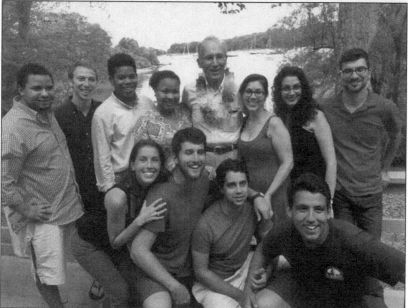

Doris and Howard with children, and Howard with grandchildren.

Howard: As I sit at my desk, I am looking for a letter that I got a couple of days ago, from Julie, my oldest grandchild the lawyer in Oakland, who spent much of a page saying how fortunate she felt to be a member of our family.

My grandchildren are pretty important to me. I am very, very lucky. These people are the children of Jon and Deborah and Fred, including the spouses of these children. They are just wonderful people. It's also a matter, to a considerable extent, of luck. My children are the treasure that fate has bestowed on me. Each chose a partner that had similar values and those in that picture who have married, chose partners with similar values.

Mark: Do you see them carrying on something important to you?

Howard: A concern for other people, that's true of all of them. So how can I look at this and not feel greatly rewarded? One of life's treasures.

Mark: We don't really realize the value of grandchildren until we have them.

Howard: I have been in a position to know that for a good deal longer than you.

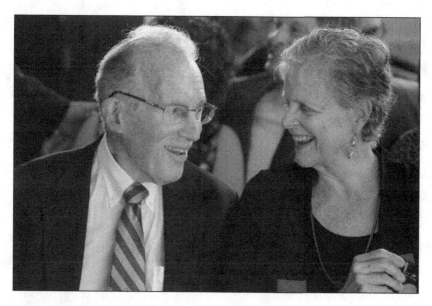

Howard and Penny.

Howard: Again, my great good fortune. I really felt that I have been fortunate to have had Doris and to have had her so long. Having lost Doris and
all that Doris meant to me, it was, again, my great good fortune that Penny
entered my life. I had known Penny for some time—she and I had worked
together on the nuclear arms issue and when I organized a program at the
academy of arts and sciences called the initiative for children. Sometime
after Doris died, Penny and I decided to come together. And that's been a
great good fortune for me. She is a very generous, caring, and good person
who focuses much of her attention on the needs of persons who are less fortunate than me. So that theme continues in the relationship. To have started
a new relationship with a new person, even though we had known each
other, but was now a relationship that differs greatly, was not easy. I think
Penny has done a great deal to make it easy. She has been far more giving
in this relationship than I have. She writes extremely well, she helped write
the memoir. She is a very caring person, she has grandchildren who are very
lucky, and she considers herself lucky for those grandchildren. And I have
had a chance to watch that and it has been rewarding.

Notes

Introduction

Philip Roth, "In Memory of a Friend, Teacher and Mentor," *New York Times*, April 20, 2013.

Chapter 1

1. Kenneth Auchincloss, "The Final Clubs: Little Bastions of Society in a University World That No Longer Cares—An Attempt to Preserve Standards of 'Gracious Living," *Harvard Crimson*, November 22, 1958.

2. David Brooks, review of Jerome Karabel, *The Chosen: The Hidden History of Admission and Exclusion at Harvard, Yale, and Princeton* (Houghton Mifflin), *New York Times*, November 6, 2005.

3. Auchincloss, "The Final Clubs."

Chapter 4

1. Robin Freedberg, interview with Howard Hiatt, *Harvard Crimson*, April 11, 1972.

2. Unsigned article, *Harvard Crimson*, May 12, 1972.

Chapter 5

1. *Boston Globe*, August 25, 1978.

Chapter 6

1. Anthony Lewis, "Abroad at Home; Thinking About the Unthinkable," *New York Times*, February 14, 1980.

2. Fox Butterfield, "Physicians Warn of Nuclear Risks,"*New York Times,* December 10, 1981.

3. "Pope to Send Out Aides in Bid to End Atomic Arms Race," *New York Times,* December 13, 1981.

4. Fox Butterfield, "Scientists' Meeting with Reagan Reflects Worry over Nuclear Peril," *New York Times,* December 18, 1981.

5. Anthony Lewis, "Hazardous to Health," *New York Times,* October 1962.

6. From Charles C. Kenney, *The Best Practice: How the New Quality Movement Is Transforming Medicine,* reprint ed..

7. Kevin Sack, "More Malpractice Than Lawsuits, New York Medical Study Suggests," *New York Times,* January 29, 1990.

8. Kevin Sack, "No-Fault for Doctors Is Called Feasible," *New York Times,* March 1, 1990.

9. Nine authors were listed for the article, "Incidence of Adverse Events and Negligence in Hospitalized Patients—Results of the Harvard Medical Practice Study," *New England Journal of Medicine* 324, no. 6 (February 7, 1991): 370–376: Troyen A. Brennan, M.P.H., M.D., J.D., Lucian L. Leape, M.D., Nan M. Laird, Ph.D., Liesi Hebert, Sc.D., A. Russell Localio, J.D., M.S., M.P.H., Ann G. Lawthers, Sc.D., Joseph P. Newhouse, Ph.D., Paul C. Weiler, LL.M., and Howard H. Hiatt, M.D.

Chapter 7

1. Howard Hiatt, "Learn from Haiti," *New York Times,* December 6, 2001.

2. Christopher Lehmann-Haupt, Review of Howard Hiatt, *America's Health in the Balance: Choice or Change? New York Times,* March 12, 1987.

3. Milt Freudenheim, "Mind/Body/Health; in Short," review of Howard Hiatt, *America's Health in the Balance: Choice or Change? New York Times,* April 5, 1987.

Chapter 9

1. Jonathan Safran Foer, *Here I Am.* New York: Farrar, Straus & Giroux, 2017.

2. Daniel Kaheneman, "Why We Contradict Ourselves and Confound Each Other," On Being podcast, October 4, 2017, https://onbeing.org/programs/daniel-kahneman -why-we-contradict-ourselves-and-confound-each-other-oct2017/

3. Rachel Yehuda, How Trauma and Resilience Cross Generations, November 9, 2017, https://onbeing.org/programs/rachel-yehuda-how-trauma-and-resilience-cross -generations/

A Life Remembered

1. Daniel Kahneman, "Why We Contradict Ourselves and Confound Each Other," interview with Krista Tippet, On Being podcast, October 4, 2017, https://onbeing .org/programs/daniel-kahneman-why-we-contradict-ourselves-and-confound-each -other-oct2017/

Index

The letter *p* following a page number denotes a photograph or information in the caption.